Emotional Stability During Menopause

Managing Anxiety, Mood Swings, and Emotional Health Throughout Perimenopause

Hillary Palms

DISCLAIMER 5

INTRODUCTION 6

CHAPTER 1: UNDERSTANDING EMOTIONAL CHANGES DURING MENOPAUSE 8

The Common Emotional Changes in Menopause 11
Menopause and Mental Health 16

CHAPTER 2: MANAGING MOOD SWINGS EFFECTIVELY IN MENOPAUSE 20

Techniques for Balancing Mood Swings in Menopause 23
Strategies to Cope with Emotional Sensitivity 31

CHAPTER 4: MENOPAUSE AND ANXIETY 42

Understanding Menopause-Related Anxiety 45
Effective Anxiety Management Techniques in menopause 50

CHAPTER 5: ALLEVIATING DEPRESSIVE SYMPTOMS 56

Recognizing Depression During Menopause 59
Techniques to Manage Depression in Menopause 64

CHAPTER 6: MENTAL HEALTH PRACTICES FOR EMOTIONAL WELL-BEING 69

Holistic Approaches to Mental Health 73
Diet and Exercise for Mental Health 77

CHAPTER 7: EMOTIONAL DETACHMENT AND RECONNECTION IN MENOPAUSE 82

Understanding Emotional Detachment in menopause 86
Reconnecting with Yourself in Menopause 90

CHAPTER 8: STRENGTHENING RELATIONSHIPS DURING MENOPAUSE 93

Navigating Emotional Challenges in Relationships 98
Maintaining Strong Relationships in Menopause 102

CHAPTER 9: COMMUNICATING EMOTIONAL NEEDS 105

TO LOVED ONES 105

Effective Communication Techniques 108
Building a Supportive Environment 112

CHAPTER 10: CRYING SPELLS AND EMOTIONAL OUTBURSTS. 117

UNDERSTANDING THE ROOT CAUSES IN MENOPAUSE 121
MANAGING SUDDEN EMOTIONAL OUTBURSTS 125

CHAPTER 11: THE EMOTIONAL ROLLERCOASTER OF MENOPAUSE 129

WHAT CAUSES THE EMOTIONAL ROLLERCOASTER? 132
BALANCING MOOD SWINGS 136

CHAPTER 12: MANAGING INCREASED ANGER AND FRUSTRATION 141

CAUSES OF MENOPAUSE-RELATED ANGER 145
TRANSFORMING ANGER INTO CALMNESS 148

CONCLUSION 152

BIOGRAPHY 153

GLOSSARY: EMOTIONAL STABILITY DURING MENOPAUSE 154

Disclaimer

The information provided in "Emotional Stability During Menopause: Managing Anxiety, Mood Swings, and Emotional Health Throughout Perimenopause" by Hillary Palms is intended for educational purposes only. This book is designed to offer general advice and insights into managing emotional health during menopause.

The content of this book should not be used as a basis for self-diagnosis or for the treatment of any health condition. Always seek the guidance of your physician or other qualified health providers with any questions you may have regarding a medical condition or treatment. Never disregard professional medical advice or delay seeking it because of something you have read in this book.

Introduction

Menopause represents a crucial transition in a woman's life, signifying the conclusion of her reproductive years and the beginning of a new phase filled with both opportunities and challenges. While it is common to associate menopause primarily with physical changes, the emotional dimensions during this period can be equally intricate and transformative.

In "Emotional Stability During Menopause," we explore the complexities of emotional health during this significant time. As women experience hormonal fluctuations, sleep disruptions, and various lifestyle adjustments that often accompany menopause, they may encounter a broad spectrum of emotions, ranging from anxiety and sadness to empowerment and renewed strength. Recognizing and comprehending these feelings is vital, as they can profoundly influence personal well-being, relationships, and everyday life.

This eBook serves as a thorough guide to achieving emotional stability during menopause, providing readers with practical strategies, insights, and support to effectively manage their emotions. Through expert guidance, personal narratives, and evidence-based methods, we aim to enhance understanding of the emotional transitions experienced during this period and offer tools to foster resilience and inner tranquility.

Whether you are nearing menopause, currently experiencing it, or supporting someone who is, this resource is crafted to empower you. We assert that grasping the emotional facets of menopause is essential for navigating this transition with poise and assurance.

Join us on this journey of self-exploration and emotional well-being as we examine the distinctive array of emotions that define menopause. Together, we will discover ways to embrace this transformative phase with optimism, strength, and stability. Welcome to a new beginning—let us embark on this enlightening journey together.

Chapter 1: Understanding Emotional Changes During Menopause

Menopause represents a crucial phase in a woman's life, signifying the conclusion of her reproductive years. Although discussions often focus on the physical manifestations, such as hot flashes, irregular menstrual cycles, and weight gain, the emotional and psychological dimensions are equally significant yet frequently neglected. This chapter seeks to illuminate the emotional transformations that accompany menopause, examining their origins, symptoms, and effects on overall well-being.

The Biological Foundation of Emotional Changes

To comprehend the emotional shifts experienced during menopause, it is essential to acknowledge the biological factors associated with this life stage. Menopause is marked by a reduction in the production of hormones, particularly estrogen and progesterone, which are vital for mood regulation and emotional health. For example, estrogen influences the synthesis of neurotransmitters such as serotonin, dopamine, and norepinephrine, all of which are crucial for maintaining emotional stability.

As hormone levels fluctuate and decrease, numerous women may face a spectrum of emotional symptoms, including mood swings, irritability, anxiety, and depression. These emotional fluctuations can be significant, creating challenges in personal relationships, professional life, and overall quality of life. The relationship between hormonal changes and emotional well-being is intricate and can be intensified by additional factors such as stress, aging, and individual life circumstances.

Common Emotional Symptoms during Menopause

Women experiencing menopause may face various emotional symptoms. Some of the most prevalent include:

Mood Swings: Similar to the emotional variations experienced during the menstrual cycle, menopause can induce intense and abrupt emotional highs and lows.

Anxiety and Panic Attacks: Many women may experience heightened anxiety, which can escalate into panic attacks, feelings of impending doom, or an inability to find relaxation.

Depression: Although not every woman will encounter depression during menopause, research suggests a significant correlation.

Psychological and Social Influences Beyond the biological factors, the emotional changes during menopause are also influenced by psychological and social elements. Many women find themselves reflecting on their lives during this phase, contemplating their identities as caregivers, professionals, and partners. The transition into menopause is often concurrent with other life changes, such as children leaving home, caring for aging parents, or approaching retirement. These experiences can exacerbate feelings of loss, anxiety, and even existential questioning.

Additionally, societal perceptions of aging and menopause can play a significant role in a woman's emotional landscape. In a culture that often idolizes youth and fertility, women may struggle with feelings of invisibility and diminished self-worth as they navigate this life stage.

Coping Mechanisms and Strategies

Understanding and addressing these emotional changes is crucial for navigating menopause with grace and resilience. Here are some strategies that can help manage emotional well-being during this time:

Open Communication: Sharing feelings with trusted friends, family, or support groups can create connections and provide a sense of belonging.

Mindfulness and Relaxation Techniques: Practices such as meditation, yoga, or deep-breathing exercises can enhance emotional regulation and reduce anxiety.

Physical Activity: Regular exercise is beneficial not only for physical health but also for mental well- being, as it can boost mood and relieve stress.

Nutritional Awareness: Maintaining a balanced diet rich in vitamins and omega-3 fatty acids can support overall mood stability.

Professional Support: Speaking with a healthcare provider or mental health professional about emotional changes can provide valuable resources, including therapy or medication if needed.

Educating Oneself: Knowledge is powerful. Understanding what to expect during menopause can help ease anxiety and empower women to approach this transition with a positive mindset.

Menopause is a multifaceted experience that encompasses not just biological changes but also profound emotional transitions. By acknowledging and understanding the emotional changes that accompany menopause, women can approach this life stage more proactively and compassionately.

The Common Emotional Changes in Menopause

While the physical symptoms of menopause, such as hot flashes and sleep disturbances, are widely known, the emotional changes that accompany this transitional period are often overlooked or misinterpreted.

Understanding the common emotional symptoms of menopause, alongside their scientific underpinnings, is crucial for women, their families, and healthcare providers to navigate this significant life stage effectively.

Understanding Menopause

Menopause itself is defined by the cessation of menstrual cycles for twelve consecutive months, primarily due to a decline in the production of hormones such as estrogen and progesterone. However, the perimenopause phase, which can start as early as a decade before menopause, is when women often first experience emotional changes. These fluctuations can vary in intensity and duration from one woman to another, influenced by genetics, lifestyle, and overall health.

Common Emotional Symptoms ### 1. Mood Swings

Many women report mood swings during perimenopause and menopause, characterized by sudden changes in emotional state. These fluctuations might include feelings of irritability, sadness, or even anger. The cause lies largely in hormonal fluctuations, which can impact the neurotransmitters that regulate mood. Reduced levels of estrogen, for instance, affect serotonin production, a neurotransmitter known for stabilizing mood.

2. Anxiety

Increased anxiety is another common emotional symptom during menopause. Women may experience generalized feelings of apprehension or specific worries about health, aging, or their roles in life. Hormonal changes, particularly a decrease in estrogen and progesterone, can alter brain chemistry and increase susceptibility to anxiety. Additionally, the psychological impact of transitioning out of childbearing years may exacerbate these feelings.

3. Depression

Some women may experience more significant depressive symptoms during menopause, which could manifest as feelings of hopelessness, loss of interest in previous activities, and fatigue. Again, hormonal fluctuations play a role, but other factors, including changes in lifestyle, relationships, and physical health, contribute to this risk. Studies suggest that these symptoms can often resolve with the restoration of hormonal balance, either through natural means or medical intervention.

4. Decreased Libido

A decline in libido during menopause can affect emotional well-being, leading to feelings of inadequacy, sadness, or anxiety about sexuality. This reduction is primarily a result of hormonal changes, but it may also stem from physical changes such as vaginal dryness and discomfort during intercourse. Open communication with partners and exploring treatment options can be beneficial in addressing these concerns.

5. Cognitive Changes

Cognitive shifts, including memory lapses and difficulty concentrating—often referred to as "brain fog"—are also common during menopause. These changes can lead to frustration or embarrassment, impacting self-esteem. Hormonal imbalances, particularly related to estrogen, have been linked to cognitive function, and further research is ongoing to fully understand this relationship.

The Science Behind Emotional Changes

The emotional changes associated with menopause underscore the complex interplay between hormones, brain chemistry, and psychosocial factors. Research indicates that estrogen has neuroprotective effects, influencing mood regulation and cognitive function. Its decline can lead to alterations in neurotransmitter systems, notably serotonin, norepinephrine, and dopamine—substances critical for mood stabilization, focus, and general emotional well-being.

Moreover, the interactions within the hypothalamic-pituitary-adrenal (HPA) axis— which regulates stress responses—can shift during menopause. Changes in hormone levels influence how the body perceives and responds to stress, potentially heightening feelings of anxiety and emotional reactivity.

Social and psychological factors also play a significant role. Changes in family dynamics, concerns about aging and health, and societal perceptions of menopause can provoke emotional distress. Women might find themselves navigating the complexities of aging while pursuing new identities beyond motherhood or professional roles, leading to an emotional reevaluation of life goals and self-worth.

Recognizing Symptoms and Seeking Support

Recognizing the emotional symptoms of menopause is the first step towards effective management and treatment. Women are encouraged to maintain open communication with healthcare providers about their experiences. Standard treatment options may include hormone replacement therapy (HRT), lifestyle modifications, and psychotherapy, aimed at addressing both the physical and emotional aspects of menopause.

Strategies for Emotional Well-Being

To support emotional well-being during menopause, women can adopt the following strategies:

Self-Care Practices: Engaging in regular physical activity, maintaining a balanced diet, and developing relaxation techniques, such as yoga or mindfulness meditation, can help manage stress and improve mood.

Social Support: Building a strong support network of friends, family, or support groups can provide emotional reassurance and help mitigate feelings of isolation.

Open Discussions: Encouraging open conversations with partners about emotional and physical changes can foster understanding and strengthen relationships.

Professional Help: Seeking therapy or counseling can be beneficial, providing a safe space to express emotions and develop coping strategies.

with confidence and clarity. Awareness, support, and informed decision-making are essential to navigating this significant life change, fostering resilience and well-being during the journey. The path through menopause can lead to new beginnings and opportunities for personal growth, reinforcing that this stage of life can be a powerful new chapter in a woman's story.

Menopause and Mental Health

While discussions surrounding menopause often emphasize its physical symptoms—such as hot flashes and vaginal dryness—the psychological and emotional aspects are equally significant. The hormonal fluctuations that occur during this stage can have a profound impact on mental health, emotional sensitivity, and overall quality of life. This chapter delves into the complex interplay between menopause, hormonal changes, and mental health, illuminating how these factors interact, their implications for emotional well-being, and effective coping strategies.

Understanding Menopause

To fully grasp the relationship between menopause and mental health, it is important to understand the nature of menopause itself. Typically occurring between the ages of 45 and 55, menopause is characterized by the end of menstruation, which results from a decrease in estrogen and progesterone levels. These hormonal changes do not occur abruptly; instead, they develop gradually over several years during a phase known as perimenopause.

As estrogen levels fluctuate and ultimately decline, various bodily systems, including the brain, undergo transformations. Estrogen is vital for the regulation of neurotransmitters, particularly serotonin and norepinephrine, which are essential for maintaining mood stability. As a result, these hormonal alterations can give rise to a range of emotional and psychological symptoms.

The Hormonal Influences on Emotions

Studies suggest that the hormonal shifts experienced

during menopause can increase vulnerability to mood disorders, anxiety, and depressive symptoms. Estrogen significantly influences the brain's chemistry and its capacity to regulate mood. Women undergoing menopause may find themselves experiencing heightened emotional sensitivity and a diminished ability to manage stress.### Anxiety and Depression

Recent studies have demonstrated that menopausal women have higher rates of anxiety and depression compared to their pre-menopausal counterparts. Anxiety symptoms may manifest as persistent worry, restlessness, or difficulty concentrating, while depressive symptoms can include feelings of worthlessness and loss of interest in previously enjoyed activities.

The interplay of hormonal changes, alongside external stressors—such as aging, changes in lifestyle, and shifts in family dynamics—can amplify these feelings. Women may feel trapped in a cycle where psychological distress feeds back into the perception of menopause itself, creating a challenging landscape for mental health.

External Factors

While hormonal changes play a critical role in emotional health during menopause, external factors must also be considered. Stressors such as caregiving responsibilities, career transitions, and health issues can compound feelings of anxiety and depression. Cultural expectations and societal attitudes toward aging can further exacerbate these emotional challenges, leading women to feel marginalized or undervalued in their later years.

Moreover, every woman's experience with menopause is unique. Individual differences, including genetics, lifestyle choices, and social support systems, contribute to how hormonal changes manifest emotionally. It's essential to recognize that while some may pass through menopause with minimal emotional disruption, others may face significant challenges requiring intervention.

Coping Strategies and Support

Given the profound link between menopause and mental health, it's crucial to explore effective coping strategies and support systems that can assist women during this transitional phase.

Lifestyle Changes

Physical Activity: Regular exercise is vital for both physical and mental health. It can boost endorphin levels, improve mood, and reduce anxiety. Engaging in activities such as walking, yoga, or dancing can foster a sense of well-being.

Nutrition: A balanced diet rich in fruits, vegetables, whole grains, and lean proteins can support overall health and help mitigate mood swings. Omega-3 fatty acids, often found in fish, have been linked to improved mood and cognitive function.

Sleep Hygiene: Sleep disturbances are common during menopause. Prioritizing sleep hygiene—establishing a regular sleep schedule, creating a restful environment, and avoiding stimulants—can aid in emotional regulation.

Mindfulness and Relaxation Techniques

Practices such as mindfulness meditation, deep breathing exercises, and progressive muscle relaxation can help women manage anxiety and improve emotional resilience.

These techniques encourage living in the moment and reducing stress, allowing for a better understanding of one's emotional responses.

Seeking Professional Help

Women experiencing significant emotional distress during menopause should not hesitate to seek professional support. Mental health professionals can provide counseling, cognitive behavioral therapy (CBT), or even medication if necessary. Educating oneself about menopause and its effects on mental health can empower women to advocate for their well-being.

Building a Support Network

Creating a robust support network can provide women with the necessary emotional encouragement during this transitional period. Friends, family, or support groups composed of women experiencing similar challenges can foster a sense of community and understanding.

The interplay of hormonal fluctuations and mental health matters deeply, influencing emotional sensitivity and overall well-being. By understanding the links between hormones and emotions, women can better navigate this transition, armed with coping strategies and the support they need.

Chapter 2: Managing Mood Swings Effectively in Menopause

One of the most frequently reported symptoms that women encounter during this transitional period is mood swings. This chapter aims to explore the nature of these emotional variations and provides practical approaches for effectively managing them.

Understanding Mood Swings During Menopause

Hormonal fluctuations significantly influence the emotional experiences associated with menopause. As estrogen levels decrease, women may face a range of symptoms, including anxiety, irritability, sadness, and even anger. These hormonal changes can affect neurotransmitters in the brain, which are essential for mood regulation. Furthermore, life changes that often accompany menopause—such as children leaving home, career transitions, or the responsibility of caring for aging parents—can intensify feelings of stress and sadness.

Common Emotional Symptoms

Mood swings during menopause can present in several ways:

Anxiety and Restlessness: Overwhelming feelings of unease or worry.

Irritability: Increased sensitivity to minor irritations or a short temper.

Depression: Ongoing feelings of sadness or hopelessness that may necessitate medical intervention.

Mood Gaps: Abrupt shifts from high to low moods without apparent cause.

It is essential to understand these symptoms as consequences of hormonal changes, life stressors, and underlying health issues. Acknowledging that mood swings are not a personal failing but rather a natural aspect of the menopausal experience can encourage women to adopt a more compassionate perspective towards themselves during this period.### 1. **Hormone Replacement Therapy (HRT)**

For some women, hormone replacement therapy can alleviate many of the emotional symptoms associated with menopause. HRT helps restore hormonal balance and can lead to significant improvements in mood. However, it's essential to discuss the potential risks and benefits with a healthcare provider to determine if HRT is the right option.

2. **Lifestyle Changes**

Lifestyle modifications can have profound effects on mood stability. Consider the following:

Regular Exercise: Engaging in physical activity releases endorphins, improves overall mood, and can be a potent antidote to anxiety and depression. Aim for at least 30 minutes of moderate exercise most days of the week.

Balanced Diet: Eating a well-balanced diet rich in fruits, vegetables, whole grains, lean proteins, and healthy fats can help stabilize energy levels and improve mood.

Hydration: Dehydration can contribute to feelings of fatigue and irritability. Drink plenty of water throughout the day to stay adequately hydrated.

Adequate Sleep: Hormonal shifts can disrupt sleep patterns. Establish a calming bedtime routine, create a comfortable sleep environment, and prioritize rest to enhance mood stability.

3. **Mindfulness and Stress Reduction**

Incorporating mindfulness practices into daily routines can greatly benefit mental health. Techniques include:

Meditation: Taking just a few minutes each day to meditate can enhance emotional regulation and decrease stress. Guided meditations, whether through apps or local classes, can provide effective structure for beginners.

Deep Breathing: Practicing deep breathing exercises can help calm the mind and reduce feelings of anxiety. Try inhaling deeply through the nose for a count of four, holding for four, and exhaling slowly through the mouth for a count of six.

Yoga and Tai Chi: These practices not only increase flexibility and physical fitness but also promote mental clarity and emotional balance.

4. **Social Support**

Strengthening connections with friends, family, or support groups can provide crucial emotional support. Sharing experiences with others can lessen feelings of isolation and offer practical strategies. Consider joining a menopause support group, either online or in-person, where members can discuss feelings, share coping strategies, and offer encouragement.

5. **Professional Help**

If mood swings become overwhelming or persist despite home remedies and lifestyle changes, it may be time to seek professional help. Mental health professionals, such as therapists or counselors, can provide coping strategies tailored to individual circumstances and, if necessary, recommend appropriate treatment options.

By understanding the interplay of hormones, stressors, and emotional well-being, women can take proactive steps to navigate this transitional phase with greater ease. Embracing the journey of menopause, with all its challenges and opportunities for growth, can lead to a more balanced and fulfilling life during and beyond this significant time.

Techniques for Balancing Mood Swings in Menopause

Among these changes, mood swings are particularly common and can be challenging to navigate. These fluctuations in mood may range from irritability and anxiety to feelings of sadness or even anger. However, evidence-based techniques such as mindfulness practices and Cognitive Behavioral Therapy (CBT) have shown great promise in managing these emotional upheavals. This chapter will explore these techniques in detail, offering insights and practical strategies that can empower women to find balance during this transitional period.

Understanding Mood Swings in Menopause

Before delving into specific techniques, it is important to understand the underlying causes of mood swings during menopause. Hormonal changes, particularly fluctuations in estrogen and progesterone, can significantly impact neurotransmitters such as serotonin and dopamine, which regulate mood. Additionally, life changes and stressors—

ranging from physical health changes to familial shifts—can contribute to emotional instability. By recognizing these contributing factors, women can better appreciate the need for effective coping strategies.

Mindfulness Practices

Mindfulness is the practice of staying present and fully engaging with the current moment, devoid of judgment. During menopause, developing mindfulness skills is particularly beneficial in managing mood swings.

1. Mindful Breathing

Mindful breathing is a fundamental technique that can be practiced anywhere. This involves focusing on the breath—inhale deeply through the nose, hold for a few seconds, and exhale slowly through the mouth. This simple act can ground individuals in the present moment, reducing anxiety and promoting relaxation.

Practical Exercise: Set aside five to ten minutes a day for mindful breathing. Create a calming space where you won't be disturbed. Close your eyes, focus on your breath, and if your mind wanders, gently guide it back to the rhythm of your breath.

2. Body Scan Meditation

The Body Scan technique involves consciously focusing on each part of the body, promoting awareness and relaxation. This practice can help women become more attuned to their physical sensations and emotional states.

Practical Exercise: Lying down in a quiet setting, systematically focus on each part of your body, starting from your toes and moving to the crown of your head. Acknowledge any sensations—tension, warmth, or relaxation—without judgment, allowing yourself to let go of stress.

3. Journaling for Mindfulness

Engaging in reflective journaling can be profoundly restorative. Writing about daily experiences, emotions, and thoughts encourages a deeper understanding of one's emotional landscape.

Practical Exercise: Dedicate a few minutes before bed to write down your thoughts and feelings of the day. Reflecting on what made you feel good and what triggered mood swings provides insight for future management.

Cognitive Behavioral Therapy (CBT)

CBT is a structured, goal-oriented psychotherapy that focuses on identifying and changing negative thought patterns and behaviors. It has proven effective for many mental health issues, including mood disorders experienced during menopause.

1. Identifying Negative Thoughts

The first step in CBT is recognizing negative thoughts that may contribute to mood swings. Common thought patterns during menopause may include "I cannot handle this" or "I'm not good enough."

Practical Exercise: Keep a thought diary where you jot down negative thoughts as they arise. Over time, this will help identify recurring patterns needing attention.

2. Challenging Cognitive Distortions

Once identified, these negative thoughts can be challenged. Consider the evidence for and against these thoughts, reframing them in a more balanced, realistic light.

Practical Exercise: For each negative thought in your diary, write down a countering thought that is more constructive or grounded in reality. For instance, if the thought is "I will never feel happy again," reframe it to "This is a challenging time, but I have experienced happiness before and can again."

3. Behavioral Activation

CBT encourages individuals to engage in activities that foster joy and fulfillment. During times of emotional distress, it can be easy to withdraw and isolate.

Practical Exercise: Create a list of enjoyable activities, whether it's pursuing a hobby, spending time with friends, or engaging in physical exercise. Schedule these activities into your week, making a commitment to engage in them even when you may not feel like it.

Combining Techniques for Optimal Results

Mindfulness and CBT are not mutually exclusive; they can be combined to create a holistic approach to managing mood swings. Incorporating mindfulness practices into the CBT framework helps foster self- awareness, enhances emotional regulation, and leads to healthier coping strategies.

Mindfulness-Integrated CBT

Consider integrating mindfulness into your CBT exercises. For instance, while working through your thought diary, practice mindful breathing to calm the mind before reflection. This combination can enhance focus, enabling deeper insight into thoughts and feelings.

Through the application of mindfulness practices and Cognitive Behavioral Therapy, individuals can cultivate tools that encourage emotional balance and resilience. As each woman embarks on her unique journey through this phase of life, embracing these techniques can empower them not only to manage mood swings but to thrive in the face of change. With practice, patience, and self-compassion, the emotional landscape of menopause can transform from a source of distress to an opportunity for growth and self- discovery.

Anticipating and Mitigating Emotional Triggers

While the focus has typically been on physical symptoms such as hot flashes and sleep disturbances, the emotional aspects deserve equal attention. This chapter explores the emotional triggers associated with menopause, discusses their implications, and offers preventative strategies to mitigate their impact. By understanding and responding to these triggers, women can navigate this life stage with greater ease and resilience.

Understanding Emotional Triggers

Emotional triggers are experiences or situations that invoke intense emotional reactions, often rooted in past experiences or current stressors. For women undergoing menopause, these triggers can be exacerbated by hormonal fluctuations, sleep disturbances, and changing life circumstances, leading to increased feelings of anxiety, sadness, or irritability.

Common Emotional Triggers During Menopause

Hormonal Changes: Fluctuations in estrogen and progesterone can influence mood-regulating neurotransmitters such as serotonin and dopamine, leading to mood swings and heightened emotional sensitivity.

Body Image Issues: Many women struggle with body image as they experience weight gain, skin changes, and other physical alterations during menopause, resulting in feelings of inadequacy and depression.

Life Transitions: Menopause often coincides with other major life transitions, such as children leaving home, aging parents, or shifts in career focus. These transitions can provoke feelings of loss, anxiety, and sadness.

Social Isolation: Research indicates that some women may withdraw socially during menopause due to mood disturbances, leading to feelings of loneliness and depression.

Sleep Disorders: Sleep disturbances common during menopause can contribute to emotional volatility, making it harder to cope with daily stressors.

Identifying Your Triggers

Identifying personal emotional triggers is the first step toward effective management. Here are some strategies to help discern specific triggers:

Journaling: Keep a daily journal to track mood changes, noting circumstances leading up to emotional peaks. Over time, patterns may emerge that highlight particular triggers.

Mood Charts: Utilize mood-tracking apps or charts to document emotional states over weeks or months, correlating them with daily activities, sleep quality, and social interactions.

Mindfulness Practices: Engage in mindfulness meditation to cultivate awareness of emotional states in real-time, helping to identify what situations or thoughts provoke strong reactions.

Feedback from Others: Speak with friends or family who may notice changes in mood or behavior. Outside perspectives can often illuminate triggers that one might overlook.

Preventative Strategies

Once triggers have been identified, preventative strategies can be deployed to mitigate their emotional effects. Below are several approaches that can empower women during this transformative phase:

1. **Lifestyle Modifications**

Regular Exercise: Physical activity is well-documented for its mood-enhancing benefits. Aim for at least 30 minutes of moderate exercise most days to boost endorphins and reduce anxiety.

Balanced Diet: Consume a nutrition-rich diet to stabilize energy levels and mood. Pay particular attention to omega-3 fatty acids, whole grains, and plenty of fruits and vegetables.

Adequate Sleep: Create a sleep-friendly environment and establish a regular sleep schedule to combat insomnia and improve emotional regulation.

2. **Relaxation Techniques**

Meditation and Yoga: Both practices enhance self-awareness and reduce stress. Incorporating these activities into your routine can cultivate a sense of calm and emotional stability.

Deep Breathing Exercises: Simple breathing techniques can help manage immediate stress responses, offering a quick way to regain composure during emotionally triggering situations.

3. **Social Support**

Communicate: Sharing feelings with supportive friends, family members, or support groups can alleviate feelings of isolation and foster connection.

Professional Counseling: Seeking therapy can offer valuable tools for managing emotions, particularly for those who experience significant distress during menopause.

4. **Education and Awareness**

Learn About Menopause: Understanding the physiological changes associated with menopause can reduce anxiety about the unknown. Educational resources, workshops, and support groups can provide valuable information and community.

5. **Mindset Shifts**

Cognitive Restructuring: Challenge negative thought patterns by reframing them in a more positive light. For example, recognize aging as a unique stage of life filled with opportunities rather than simply a loss of youth.

Gratitude Practice: Cultivating a habit of gratitude can shift focus away from negative emotions, fostering resilience and a more positive outlook.

By identifying personal triggers and engaging in preventative measures, women can navigate the emotional landscape of menopause with greater confidence and equanimity. This chapter aims to empower women to embrace this natural transition, fostering emotional well-being and resilience through understanding and preparation. Ultimately, by taking charge of emotional health during menopause, women can emerge stronger and more self-aware, ready to embrace the next chapter of their lives with grace and vigor.

Strategies to Cope with Emotional Sensitivity
Emotional sensitivity can present significant challenges during menopause. This chapter seeks to provide readers with practical approaches to managing emotional sensitivity, emphasizing effective self-care techniques and the value of established support systems.

Comprehending Emotional Sensitivity
As hormonal levels fluctuate throughout menopause, women may encounter increased emotional sensitivity, which can manifest as anxiety, mood fluctuations, irritability, or feelings of sadness. This emotional turmoil is often a natural result of the biological changes taking place within the body. It is essential to recognize these emotions without judgment to manage them effectively.

The Biological Foundations of Emotional Sensitivity

Gaining insight into the physiological aspects of emotional sensitivity can empower women to view their feelings as normal reactions to hormonal changes. The decline of estrogen during menopause significantly affects mood regulation, potentially leading to mood disturbances. Furthermore, as women age and experience lifestyle changes, they may encounter additional stressors, such as caregiving duties or career shifts, which can exacerbate emotional fluctuations. Acknowledging these influences is a crucial step in developing effective coping strategies.

Self-Care Strategies for Managing Emotional Sensitivity During Menopause

Engaging in self-care is vital for addressing emotional sensitivity during menopause. The following strategies can bolster emotional resilience and enhance overall well-being.

1. Mindfulness and Meditation

Mindfulness entails being fully present and observing one's thoughts and feelings without criticism. Engaging in simple mindfulness practices, such as concentrating on one's breath or participating in guided meditation, can alleviate anxiety and facilitate emotional recovery. It is beneficial to allocate a few minutes each day to mindfulness exercises, creating an opportunity for emotional processing and grounding.### 2. Physical Activity

Regular physical activity is not only beneficial for physical health but also acts as a powerful mood enhancer. Exercise releases endorphins, which can improve mood and decrease feelings of anxiety and depression. Whether through yoga, walking, dancing, or any preferred activity, find enjoyable ways to incorporate movement into daily routines.

3. Nutritional Awareness

Studies have shown that there is a solid link between diet and emotional health. Incorporating a diet rich in omega-3 fatty acids, whole grains, fruits, and vegetables can support overall well-being. Staying hydrated and limiting caffeine and alcohol can also play significant roles in mood stability. Consider consulting with a nutritionist or dietitian to tailor dietary choices to individual needs.

4. Creative Expression

Engaging in creative activities can serve as an emotional outlet. Whether through painting, writing, music, or crafting, the process of creating can be cathartic and provide clarity. Making time for hobbies you are passionate about can release pent-up emotions and serve as a healthy way to process feelings.

5. Journaling

Writing about one's feelings and experiences can provide insight into emotional states, helping to identify patterns and triggers. Starting a journaling practice can serve as a safe space for reflection, allowing for deeper understanding and acceptance of emotional sensitivity.

Building Support Networks

Community is vital during challenging times. The significance of connection and support cannot be overstated, as shared experiences and understanding can foster resilience.

1. Family Support

Engage with family members about the emotional changes you may be experiencing. Open communication can create an empathetic atmosphere where family members understand the challenges faced and can offer support in various ways.

2. Friends and Peer Groups

Forming or joining a support group, either in person or online, provides a platform to share experiences and gain insights from others undergoing similar transitions. Group sessions—facilitated by a professional or peer-led—can offer collective wisdom, encouragement, and emotional support.

3. Professional Counseling

In some instances, emotional sensitivity could benefit from professional support. A therapist specializing in menopause or women's health can provide techniques tailored to your needs, empowering you to manage emotional sensitivities more effectively.

4. Educational Workshops

Consider attending workshops focused on menopause and emotional well-being. These can provide valuable tools, resources, and connection with others navigating the same experiences. Many organizations offer online courses or webinars that can be accessed remotely.

Embracing the Journey

It is essential for women experiencing menopause to remember that sensitivity, while challenging, is part of a natural process. Embracing this journey requires acknowledgment, self-compassion, and a willingness to seek out the tools that will create a supportive environment.

This chapter emphasizes the importance of self-care and establishing strong support networks to navigate emotional sensitivity during menopause. By integrating these strategies into daily life, women can cultivate a deeper understanding of themselves and emerge from this life stage with resilience and strength.

As we move forward, remember: you are not alone, and the path through menopause can be navigated successfully with the right tools and support systems in place. Let this chapter serve as a guide to help you flourish during this transformative time in your life.

Creating a Calming Environment

Hot flashes, sleep disturbances, mood fluctuations, and fatigue are prevalent symptoms that can interfere with both domestic life and professional performance. Establishing a serene environment—at home and in the workplace—can greatly ease the difficulties associated with these symptoms. This chapter delves into practical modifications to your surroundings and presents various relaxation strategies that can cultivate a sense of calm and well-being during this significant transition.

1. Recognizing the Influence of Environment
The environments we occupy significantly impact our mood, energy, and overall health. For women experiencing menopause, an atmosphere that encourages comfort and serenity is essential. It is important to

identify factors that may induce stress or worsen symptoms, such as disorganization, loud noises, or uncomfortable temperatures, and take proactive measures to address them.

1.1 The Significance of Personal Comfort
Customization is crucial in establishing a relaxing environment. Women should feel encouraged to design their spaces in a way that reflects their tastes and fosters relaxation. Minor adjustments can greatly enhance the welcoming nature of a space and reduce stress.

2. Modifications at Home for a Tranquil Environment
2.1 Managing Temperature
Temperature variations are a common aspect of menopause. Maintaining a cool environment is vital for alleviating hot flashes, so consider implementing the following changes:

Install a Programmable Thermostat:
Utilize a programmable thermostat to ensure a comfortable temperature in your home. Set it to cooler levels during the night to promote improved sleep quality.

Utilize Fans Effectively:
Ceiling fans, standing fans, or portable fans can efficiently circulate air. Position a fan near your sleeping area or workspace to provide a refreshing breeze during episodes of hot flashes.**Cooling Bedding:**

Invest in breathable, moisture-wicking bedding materials like cotton or bamboo to help regulate body temperature while sleeping.

2.2 Creating Relaxing Spaces

Designated relaxation zones in the home can serve as retreats from daily stressors. Consider establishing spaces dedicated to self-care:

Comfortable Seating:

Invest in a cozy chair or lounge area where you can read, meditate, or unwind. Add soft cushions and perhaps a weighted blanket for added comfort.

Nature Indoors:

Incorporating plants can significantly enhance your indoor environment. They improve air quality and bring a sense of tranquility. Look for low-maintenance varieties like peace lilies or snake plants.

Soft Lighting:

Dim lighting can foster a calming atmosphere. Use warm LED bulbs, fairy lights, or table lamps to create a soothing ambiance in your home.

2.3 Decluttering

A cluttered space can lead to a cluttered mind. Taking the time to organize and declutter can have a significant positive effect on your mental health:

Minimalist Approach:

Adopt a minimalist mindset. Keep only items that bring you joy or serve a purpose.

Create a Daily Routine:

Incorporate a few minutes each day to tidy up. Maintaining order can reduce anxiety and make your space feel more serene.

3. Workplace Adjustments for a Supportive Environment

For many women experiencing menopause, the workplace can be an additional source of stress. Making thoughtful adjustments can lead to a more accommodating and less distracting environment.

3.1 Flexible Working Arrangements

A supportive employer can make a significant difference. If possible, consider the following:

Remote Work Options:

If your job allows, opt for remote work on days when symptoms may be more pronounced. This can provide relief from commuting and office temperature variations.

Flexible Hours:

Discuss the possibility of flexible working hours with your employer. Finding a schedule that aligns with your peak productivity and comfort can aid in managing symptoms more effectively.

3.2 Ergonomic Workstation Setup

Creating a comfortable and ergonomically sound workspace can make long hours at a desk more manageable:

Adjustable Chair and Desk:

Ensure that your chair provides good support and that your desk is at an appropriate height to prevent strain.

Personal Climate Controls:

Consider using a personal fan or space heater, depending on your sensitivity to temperature changes. ### 3.3 Stress-Relief Options

Many workplaces are beginning to acknowledge the importance of mental health, and simple stress-relief options can be helpful:

Designated Break Areas:

Encourage the use of break rooms equipped with comfortable seating, soothing colors, and—if possible—green plants.

Quiet Zones:

Establish areas where employees can retreat for quiet time or meditation, even if just for a few minutes. ## 4. Relaxation Techniques for Managing Symptoms

In addition to environmental adjustments, incorporating relaxation techniques into your daily routine can provide significant relief from menopause symptoms.

4.1 Mindfulness and Meditation

Practicing mindfulness and meditation can help reduce stress and anxiety:

Breath Awareness:

Take a few moments each day to focus solely on your breath. Inhale deeply through your nose, hold for a few seconds, and exhale smoothly. This simple practice can center your mind and reduce feelings of overwhelm.

Guided Meditation:

Utilize mobile apps or online resources for guided meditation sessions. Aim for 10-15 minutes per day, particularly during stressful moments.

4.2 Exercise and Movement

Regular physical activity is essential for emotional and physical well-being:

Low-Impact Activities:

Consider yoga, swimming, or walking as gentle forms of exercise that can reduce stress and improve mood.

Stretching Routines:

Incorporate gentle stretching exercises throughout your day to release physical tension and improve circulation.

4.3 Aromatherapy

Utilizing essential oils can create a calming environment:

Diffusers:

Use an essential oil diffuser with calming scents such as lavender, chamomile, or bergamot. These scents can promote relaxation and help alleviate anxiety.

Bath Rituals:

Incorporate essential oils into your bath for a soothing experience to unwind at the end of the day. ### 4.4 Journaling

Putting thoughts and feelings onto paper can be a powerful outlet:

Gratitude Journals:

Keep a gratitude journal to reflect on positive moments each day. This simple practice can shift your focus away from stress and promote a more optimistic mindset.

Emotional Releases:

Write down any worries or feelings to help process and release them, providing clarity during turbulent times.

Remember, this is a time of transition, and embracing the changes with intentionality and compassion towards yourself can significantly enhance your quality of life. By taking proactive steps to create calm, you equip yourself to not only endure but thrive during this pivotal chapter. Empower yourself to cultivate tranquility, and you'll likely find that you can face the challenges of menopause with renewed strength and resilience.

Chapter 4: Menopause and Anxiety

While the physical manifestations of menopause—such as hot flashes, night sweats, and fluctuations in weight—are often highlighted, the psychological ramifications tend to be overlooked. Anxiety, a prevalent yet frequently underestimated aspect of menopause, can be significantly influenced by this transitional phase.

Understanding Menopause

Menopause generally occurs between the ages of 45 and 55, initiated by a notable decrease in hormone production, particularly estrogen and progesterone. This hormonal decline not only affects physical health but also has repercussions on mood and emotional stability. For numerous women, this period can trigger feelings of loss related to fertility, aging, and personal identity, all of which may contribute to increased anxiety.

Hormonal Changes and Mood

Estrogen directly influences neurotransmitters in the brain, including serotonin, which is crucial for mood regulation. The decrease in estrogen levels during menopause can result in mood fluctuations, irritability, and heightened anxiety. Research indicates that women may experience a worsening of pre-existing anxiety disorders during this time, as hormonal changes can intensify feelings of discomfort and panic.

Moreover, progesterone is recognized for its soothing properties; it aids in promoting sleep and alleviating anxiety. As the levels of these hormones vary, women's capacity to manage stress may be diminished, creating a cyclical relationship where anxiety leads to insomnia, which in turn exacerbates anxiety.

The Psychological Landscape of Menopause

Cultural narratives surrounding menopause can significantly influence how women navigate this transition. Societal norms often associate aging and menopause with negative implications, such as reduced desirability, loss of youth, or a decline in femininity.

These societal perceptions can heighten feelings of anxiety and self-doubt, trapping women in a cycle of comparison and insecurity. Moreover, the transition into menopause may coincide with other life stressors, such as caring for aging parents, navigating changes in one's career, or experiencing shifts in personal relationships. This multifaceted stress can create a perfect storm that propels anxiety to the forefront of a woman's emotional landscape.

Identifying Anxiety Symptoms

Recognizing anxiety during menopause is essential for effective management. Symptoms may include:

Persistent worry or fear: Feeling a sense of doom or lingering unease without a clear cause.

Physical symptoms: Increased heart rate, muscle tension, fatigue, or gastrointestinal disturbances.

Sleep disturbances: Difficulty falling asleep, staying asleep, or experiencing restless nights.

Cognitive changes: Difficulty with concentration, memory lapses, or a feeling of being overwhelmed.

For many women, these symptoms may be misattributed

to normal aging or dismissed as simply part of menopause. However, acknowledging and addressing such feelings is crucial for mental well-being.

Coping Mechanisms and Solutions

Fortunately, there are several strategies to help manage anxiety during menopause. Each woman's experience is unique, and a combination of approaches may be necessary to achieve relief:

Therapy and Counseling: Engaging with a mental health professional can provide support and coping strategies. Cognitive-behavioral therapy (CBT) is particularly effective for anxiety disorders, enabling women to reframe their thoughts and develop healthier coping mechanisms.

Medication: For some women, medication may be necessary to manage anxiety effectively. Options can include antidepressants or hormone replacement therapy (HRT), which may help alleviate both physical and psychological symptoms.

Lifestyle Changes: Incorporating regular exercise, a balanced diet, and adequate sleep can significantly improve mood and reduce anxiety levels. Activities such as yoga and meditation have also been shown to promote relaxation and alleviate stress.

Social Support: Connecting with friends, family, or support groups can counter feelings of isolation. Shared experiences can foster solidarity and provide a safe space to express concerns.

Mindfulness and Relaxation Techniques: Practicing mindfulness can help women stay grounded and present, reducing anxiety's grip. Techniques such as deep breathing, progressive muscle relaxation, or guided imagery can encourage a sense of calm.

Moving Forward

It's essential to create an open dialogue about menopause and mental health. Women should feel empowered to discuss their experiences with healthcare providers, exploring treatments and coping strategies that work best for them. By addressing anxiety as a legitimate and treatable aspect of menopause, women can reclaim their narrative and navigate this transition with greater assurance and resilience.

Menopause is a significant life change that can bring forth a complex interplay of emotions. While anxiety can accompany this phase, understanding its roots, recognizing symptoms, and implementing effective coping strategies can lead to a healthier, more balanced transition. Women deserve support and resources to manage their mental health alongside the physical challenges posed by menopause, allowing them to thrive in this new chapter of life.

Understanding Menopause-Related Anxiety

While the physical manifestations of menopause—such as hot flashes, night sweats, and fluctuations in weight—are often highlighted, the psychological ramifications tend to be overlooked. Anxiety, a prevalent yet frequently underestimated aspect of menopause, can be significantly influenced by this transitional phase.

Understanding Menopause
Menopause generally occurs between the ages of 45 and 55, initiated by a notable decrease in hormone production, particularly estrogen and progesterone. This hormonal decline not only affects physical health but also has repercussions on mood and emotional stability. For numerous women, this period can trigger feelings of loss related to fertility, aging, and personal identity, all of which may contribute to increased anxiety.

Hormonal Changes and Mood
Estrogen directly influences neurotransmitters in the brain, including serotonin, which is crucial for mood regulation. The decrease in estrogen levels during menopause can result in mood fluctuations, irritability, and heightened anxiety. Research indicates that women may experience a worsening of pre-existing anxiety disorders during this time, as hormonal changes can intensify feelings of discomfort and panic.

Moreover, progesterone is recognized for its soothing properties; it aids in promoting sleep and alleviating anxiety. As the levels of these hormones vary, women's capacity to manage stress may be diminished, creating a cyclical relationship where anxiety leads to insomnia, which in turn exacerbates anxiety.

The Psychological Landscape of Menopause
Cultural narratives surrounding menopause can significantly influence how women navigate this transition. Societal norms often associate aging and menopause with negative implications, such as reduced

desirability, loss of youth, or a decline in femininity. These societal perceptions can heighten feelings of anxiety and self-doubt, trapping women in a cycle of comparison and insecurity.

Causes of Menopause-Related Anxiety ### Biological Factors

The primary biological cause of menopause-related anxiety is hormonal fluctuation. The dramatic and rapid changes in hormone levels can disrupt the balance of neurotransmitters, leading to mood disorders. Also, genetics may play a part; women with a history of anxiety or mood disorder in their families may be more susceptible to anxiety during menopause.

Psychological Factors

The transition into menopause can also force women to confront many psychological challenges. This period is often associated with various life changes—such as aging, shifting roles in the family, or approaching retirement—that can stir feelings of loss and uncertainty. The anticipation of these changes, combined with physical symptoms, can exacerbate feelings of anxiety.

Lifestyle Factors

Lifestyle choices made by women before and during menopause may also influence anxiety levels. High-stress lifestyles, poor diet, lack of exercise, and inadequate sleep can significantly heighten anxiety symptoms. Moreover, substance use, including alcohol and caffeine, can contribute to anxiety and must be monitored during this transitional phase.

Symptoms of Menopause-Related Anxiety

Recognizing the symptoms of menopause-related anxiety is crucial for managing mental health effectively. The symptoms can vary widely from woman to woman but commonly include:

Persistent Worry: An overwhelming sense of dread or persistent worry about health, relationships, career, and other life events.

Physical Symptoms: Increased heart rate, sweating, trembling, and gastrointestinal disturbances can occur alongside psychological symptoms.

Mood Swings: Unpredictable emotional fluctuations may manifest, leading to irritability, sadness, or frustration.

Sleep Disturbances: Insomnia or disrupted sleep is common during menopause, exacerbating feelings of anxiety.

Difficulty Concentrating: Many women report experiencing 'brain fog,' making it challenging to focus or make decisions.

Social Withdrawal: A tendency to avoid social situations or isolate oneself due to anxiety can further impact mental health.

Coping Strategies and Treatment Options

Understanding the link between hormonal changes and anxiety allows women to take proactive steps in managing their mental health. Here are several strategies and treatments that may alleviate menopause- related anxiety:

Lifestyle Modifications

Exercise: Regular physical activity has been proven to reduce anxiety and improve mood. A combination of aerobic exercise, strength training, and relaxation techniques such as yoga or tai chi can be especially beneficial.

Nutrition: A balanced diet rich in whole foods, omega-3 fatty acids, and antioxidants has been shown to support brain health and mood regulation. Reducing caffeine and alcohol consumption can also help manage anxiety symptoms.

Sleep Hygiene: Prioritizing sleep through improved habits can significantly reduce anxiety. Establishing a calming bedtime routine and creating a restful sleep environment are essential.

Psychological Interventions

Cognitive Behavioral Therapy (CBT): This evidence-based therapy can help women reframe negative thought patterns associated with anxiety and develop coping strategies.

Mindfulness and Relaxation Techniques: Practices such as meditation and deep-breathing exercises can promote relaxation and reduce symptoms of anxiety.

Hormonal and Non-Hormonal Treatments

Hormone replacement therapy (HRT) may provide relief for some women by restoring hormonal balance. However, it is essential to discuss the potential risks and benefits with a healthcare provider. Non-hormonal medications, such as selective serotonin reuptake inhibitors (SSRIs), may also be prescribed for anxiety management.

The anxiety many women experience during this time can be closely linked to hormonal changes affecting mood and emotional well-being. By understanding the relationship between these changes and anxiety, women can take actionable steps to manage their symptoms and seek appropriate support. Creating an open dialogue about menopause-related anxiety is crucial to breaking the stigma surrounding this natural phase of life, ultimately empowering women to navigate their experiences with confidence and resilience.

Effective Anxiety Management Techniques in menopause

Fluctuating hormone levels can intensify feelings of stress, irritability, and anxiety, thereby affecting daily activities and overall health. Gaining an understanding of and adopting effective anxiety management strategies, such as relaxation techniques, medications, and natural remedies, can enable women to navigate this transitional period with increased ease and assurance.

Understanding Anxiety in Menopause ### The Biological Basis

During menopause, there is a decline in estrogen and progesterone levels, which can affect the neurotransmitter systems in the brain that regulate mood. Reduced estrogen levels may result in heightened sensitivity to stress and increased anxiety. This biological change, combined with external stressors such as aging, caregiving responsibilities, or significant life transitions, can create a challenging environment for anxiety.

Psychological Factors
From a psychological perspective, the transition through menopause may evoke feelings of loss related to fertility, youth, or personal identity. Such emotions can exacerbate anxiety, highlighting the necessity for effective management techniques.

Relaxation Exercises ### 1. Deep Breathing
Deep breathing techniques serve as straightforward yet effective methods for alleviating anxiety. They function by triggering the body's relaxation response.
How to Practice Deep Breathing:
Locate a quiet area and sit or lie down in a comfortable position.
Inhale deeply through your nose, allowing your abdomen to expand.
Pause for a moment while holding your breath.
Exhale slowly through your mouth.

Continue this process for several minutes, concentrating on the rhythm of your breathing. ### 2. Progressive Muscle Relaxation (PMR)

PMR entails the methodical tensing and relaxing of various muscle groups to alleviate physical tension and anxiety.**How to Practice PMR:**

Begin with your feet; tense the muscles for a count of five, then release.

Move to your calves, thighs, abdomen, arms, shoulders, and face, repeating the tensing and relaxing process.

Pay attention to the difference between tension and relaxation in each muscle group. ### 3. Mindfulness Meditation Mindfulness meditation encourages being present in the moment, reducing worries about the future or regrets about the past.

How to Practice Mindfulness:

Sit in a comfortable position with your eyes closed.

Focus on your breath, noticing each inhale and exhale.

When thoughts arise, acknowledge them without judgment, letting them drift away.

Aim for ten to fifteen minutes of mindfulness practice daily. ### 4. Yoga

Yoga not only improves flexibility and strength but also promotes relaxation and stress relief.

How to Start Yoga:

Join a local class or follow online tutorials tailored for beginners.

Focus on gentle, restorative yoga poses that emphasize breathing and mindfulness.

Incorporate poses like Child's Pose, Cat-Cow, and Corpse Pose. ## Medications

1. Hormone Replacement Therapy (HRT)

HRT can alleviate menopausal symptoms, including anxiety. By restoring hormonal balance, it can help reduce mood swings and anxiety levels. Consult a healthcare provider to discuss the risks and benefits based on individual health history.

2. Antidepressants and Anti-Anxiety Medications

Selective serotonin reuptake inhibitors (SSRIs) and other medications prescribed for anxiety and depression may also be effective for menopause-related anxiety. These medications help regulate mood and manage anxiety symptoms but should always be used under professional supervision.

Natural Remedies

1. Herbal Supplements

Certain herbal remedies can support emotional well-being. Popular options include:

St. John's Wort: Used for mild to moderate depression.

Valerian Root: Known for promoting relaxation and reducing anxiety.

Ginseng: May improve mood and combat fatigue.

Always consult a healthcare provider before starting any herbal regimen, as interactions with other medications may occur.

2. Dietary Considerations

A balanced diet plays a vital role in emotional health. Key components include:

Omega-3 Fatty Acids: Found in fish, flaxseed, and walnuts; they support brain health.

Whole Grains and Complex Carbohydrates: Help maintain stable blood sugar levels and improve mood.

Hydration: Proper hydration supports overall health and can influence mood and mental clarity. ### 3. Regular Exercise Physical activity is a powerful anxiety management tool. Engaging in regular exercise releases endorphins, the body's natural mood lifters.

Recommended Activities:

Walking or jogging

Swimming

Dancing

Cycling

Aim for at least 150 minutes of moderate aerobic activity weekly.

By employing effective anxiety management techniques such as relaxation exercises, considering medications, and utilizing natural remedies, women can enhance their emotional and psychological resilience during this transformative phase.

Chapter 5: Alleviating Depressive Symptoms

This chapter will examine various strategies to alleviate these symptoms, offering a thorough overview of both lifestyle changes and medical treatments that can assist women during this difficult period.

Understanding Depressive Symptoms During Menopause

Menopause generally occurs between the ages of 45 and 55; however, the transition leading up to it, referred to as perimenopause, may commence several years prior. The fluctuations in estrogen levels can result in a range of psychological symptoms, including feelings of sadness, anxiety, irritability, and mood fluctuations. The likelihood of experiencing significant depression also rises during this phase, influenced by factors such as age, stress levels, personal history of depression, and shifts in life circumstances.

It is essential to acknowledge that depressive symptoms are legitimate and warrant attention; they should not be dismissed as merely a natural aspect of aging or menopausal transitions. Recognizing these symptoms can empower women to seek assistance and validate their experiences.

Lifestyle Modifications
Regular Physical Activity:
Participating in consistent exercise is among the most effective natural approaches to mitigating depressive symptoms. Aerobic activities, such as walking, swimming,

or cycling, can enhance the production of endorphins—hormones that function as natural mood lifters. Furthermore, practices like yoga and tai chi foster mindfulness and relaxation, yielding both physical and emotional advantages.

Balanced Nutrition:
A nutritious diet can profoundly influence mood and energy levels. Including nutrient-dense foods such as fruits, vegetables, whole grains, lean proteins, and healthy fats can provide essential support for mental well-being. Omega-3 fatty acids, prevalent in fish and flaxseeds, have been associated with a decreased risk of depression. Maintaining proper hydration and moderating caffeine and alcohol intake is also advantageous, as these substances can intensify mood swings and anxiety.

Sleep Hygiene:
Sleep disturbances are common during menopause, and poor sleep can exacerbate depressive symptoms. Establishing a consistent sleep schedule, creating a calming bedtime routine, and ensuring a comfortable sleep environment can help improve sleep quality. Techniques such as deep breathing exercises or progressive muscle relaxation may also aid in reducing anxiety related to sleep.

Mindfulness and Stress Reduction:

Mindfulness practices such as meditation, deep-breathing exercises, and mindfulness-based cognitive therapy can help women manage stress and cultivate a sense of calm. Engaging in creative outlets, such as painting, writing, or gardening, can provide a therapeutic way to express emotions and relieve stress.

Social Support:

Connecting with friends, family, or support groups can provide an invaluable emotional outlet. Sharing experiences with others who are going through similar challenges can foster a sense of community and understanding. Women are encouraged to seek out support, whether through informal gatherings or organized groups focused on women's health during menopause.

Medical Interventions

While lifestyle modifications can be highly effective, some women may require additional support through medical interventions:

Hormone Replacement Therapy (HRT):

HRT can help stabilize hormone levels, leading to a reduction in both physical and emotional menopausal symptoms. It is essential for women to discuss the potential benefits and risks of HRT with their healthcare provider to determine whether it is the right option for them.

Antidepressant Medications:

Selective serotonin reuptake inhibitors (SSRIs) and other antidepressants may be prescribed to alleviate depressive symptoms, especially in women who have a history of depression. These medications can help in balancing neurotransmitters that affect mood.

Cognitive Behavioral Therapy (CBT):

CBT has proven effective in treating depressive symptoms

by addressing negative thought patterns and behaviors. This form of therapy can provide women with practical tools to cope with mood changes and mental distress during menopause.

Alternative Therapies:

Some women may find relief through alternative therapies such as acupuncture, herbal supplements, or homeopathy. However, it is crucial to discuss these options with a healthcare professional, as not all alternative treatments are suitable for everyone.

Navigating the emotional landscape of menopause can be challenging, but understanding and addressing depressive symptoms is vital for overall well-being. By incorporating lifestyle changes, seeking social support, and exploring medical options, women can effectively alleviate depressive symptoms.

Recognizing Depression During Menopause

While it's often discussed in terms of hot flashes and night sweats, menopause can also significantly impact mental health, leading to an increased risk of depression. Recognizing the symptoms of depression during this time, understanding the diagnosis process, and navigating the emotional rollercoaster can empower women to seek help and embrace this new phase of life with resilience.

Understanding Menopause and Its Impact on Mental Health

Menopause typically occurs between the ages of 45 and 55, although it can happen earlier due to surgical procedures or medical conditions. The hormonal fluctuations that accompany menopause—most notably a decrease in estrogen and progesterone—can affect neurotransmitters in the brain, such as serotonin and norepinephrine, which are critical for mood regulation. Consequently, this period of hormonal change can heighten a woman's vulnerability to depression.

Common Symptoms of Depression During Menopause

Awareness of the specific symptoms of depression during menopause is essential for timely intervention. Symptoms can vary widely and may include:

Emotional Symptoms:

Persistent feelings of sadness or emptiness

Increased irritability or frustration

Anxiety and worries about health, relationships, or the future

Feelings of hopelessness or helplessness

Loss of interest in previously enjoyed activities

Physical Symptoms:

Fatigue or low energy levels

Changes in sleep patterns, including insomnia or hypersomnia

Appetite changes, including overeating or loss of appetite

Difficulty concentrating or making decisions

Somatic complaints, which may include headaches or gastrointestinal issues

Cognitive Symptoms:

Trouble focusing or memory lapses

Overwhelming feelings of stress or being overstimulated

Indecision or experiencing mental fog

Behavioral Symptoms:

Withdrawal from friends and loved ones

Increased reliance on alcohol or other substances

Neglecting responsibilities at home or work

It is crucial to recognize that not every woman will experience these symptoms with the same intensity or combination. Furthermore, many women may dismiss their emotional struggles as a normal response to aging or life changes, delaying the recognition of underlying depression.

The Diagnosis Process

If a woman suspects she might be experiencing depression during menopause, consulting a healthcare provider is an essential step. Diagnosis typically involves:

Comprehensive Assessment:

Healthcare providers will assess physical health, personal and family medical history, and psychological symptoms. Instruments like depression screening questionnaires may be utilized.

Rule Out Other Conditions:

It is vital to differentiate depression from other medical issues such as thyroid dysfunction, anemia, or chronic illness, which can present similar symptoms.

Assessment of Hormonal Changes:

Sometimes, measuring hormone levels can be informative, although the relationship between hormone changes and mental health can be complex and individual.

Psychological Evaluations:

Mental health professionals may employ clinical interviews and standardized tests to better evaluate the presence and severity of depressive symptoms.

Recognizing depression early on increases the likelihood of successful treatment, allowing women to reclaim their mental wellbeing.

Riding the Emotional Rollercoaster

Menopause can feel like an emotional rollercoaster, with various highs and lows frequently tied to fluctuating hormone levels. Here, it's vital to acknowledge that experiencing intense emotions—like mood swings, irritability, and even irrational emotional responses—is not uncommon. Many women find themselves navigating periods of joy, frustration, sadness, and anxiety that can feel overwhelming.

Coping Mechanisms:

Practicing mindfulness and meditation can assist women in managing their emotions and finding centers of calm amidst chaos.

Engaging in regular physical activity is known to release endorphins, which can enhance mood and energy.

Seeking social support, whether from friends, family, or support groups, can provide reassurance and understanding during this tumultuous time.

Professional Support:

For some, therapy can offer tools to comprehend their emotions more deeply and develop strategies to cope with and manage symptoms of depression. Cognitive Behavioral Therapy (CBT) has shown effectiveness in many cases.

Medical Interventions:

In some instances, hormone replacement therapy (HRT) or antidepressant medications may be recommended to alleviate both menopausal symptoms and depressive symptoms.

Reframing the Experience:

While it may feel impossible at times, reframing menopause as a new chapter rather than an end can inspire resilience. Embracing change—acknowledging its challenges but focusing on personal growth—can serve to empower women during this transitional phase.

Techniques to Manage Depression in Menopause
Menopause may provide relief from the challenges associated with menstruation; however, it can also introduce a range of emotional difficulties, including depression. This chapter seeks to examine effective therapeutic strategies and lifestyle modifications that can assist in managing depression during menopause, emphasizing a comprehensive approach to mental and emotional health.

Understanding Depression in Menopause
Menopause is characterized by the cessation of menstrual cycles for a minimum of 12 consecutive months, typically occurring between the ages of 45 and 55. This transitional period is often marked by various symptoms, such as hot flashes, sleep disturbances, and mood fluctuations. The hormonal changes that occur during menopause, particularly the reduction in estrogen and progesterone levels, can intensify feelings of sadness and anxiety, thereby increasing the likelihood of depression.

Recognizing Symptoms of Depression
Prior to exploring management strategies, it is crucial to identify the symptoms of depression, which can manifest differently in each individual. Common indicators include:
- Persistent feelings of sadness or low mood
- Diminished interest in previously enjoyed activities
- Alterations in appetite or weight
- Sleep disturbances, such as insomnia or excessive sleeping
- Difficulty with concentration
- Feelings of worthlessness or overwhelming guilt
- Fatigue or a lack of energy

- Thoughts of death or suicide

Early recognition of these symptoms can facilitate more effective management and treatment options.

Therapeutic Options

1. Psychotherapy

Psychotherapy, commonly referred to as talk therapy, can serve as a valuable intervention for addressing depression during menopause. Cognitive-behavioral therapy (CBT) is particularly advantageous, as it aims to identify and modify negative thought patterns and behaviors. In addition to CBT, supportive therapy and group therapy can offer emotional support and foster a sense of community, enabling women to navigate this transitional period with enhanced resilience.### 2. Pharmacotherapy

For some women, medication may be necessary to manage moderate to severe depression. Antidepressants, particularly selective serotonin reuptake inhibitors (SSRIs), have proven effective in treating menopause-related depression. Moreover, hormone replacement therapy (HRT) may also be considered for those experiencing severe menopausal symptoms, as it can help stabilize mood and alleviate depressive symptoms. It is crucial to consult with a healthcare provider to evaluate the risks and benefits of any medication.

3. Mindfulness and Meditation

Mindfulness practices and meditation have gained popularity as therapeutic approaches for managing mental health. These techniques encourage individuals to focus on the present moment, promoting relaxation and reducing anxiety. Regular practice can help women better cope with the emotional changes associated with menopause.

4. Support Groups

Peer support is invaluable during menopause. Support groups provide a space for women to share experiences, strategies, and encouragement. Joining a community of like-minded individuals can reduce feelings of isolation and foster a sense of belonging.

Lifestyle Changes

In addition to therapeutic options, certain lifestyle changes can play a significant role in managing depression during menopause.

1. Nutrition

A well-balanced diet rich in fruits, vegetables, whole grains, and lean proteins can positively affect mood and energy levels. Omega-3 fatty acids, found in fish, flaxseeds, and walnuts, have been linked to improved mental health. Limiting caffeine and alcohol can also help stabilize mood and reduce anxiety.

2. Physical Activity

Regular physical exercise is one of the most effective strategies for managing depression. Exercise releases endorphins, the body's natural mood elevators, and can significantly reduce feelings of sadness. Aim for at least 30 minutes of moderate exercise most days of the week. Walking, swimming, and yoga are excellent options that cater to different fitness levels.

3. Sleep Hygiene

Adequate sleep is crucial for mental health. Developing a consistent sleep routine, creating a calming bedtime environment, and practicing relaxation techniques can improve sleep quality. If sleep disturbances persist, seeking medical advice is essential.

4. Stress Management

Chronic stress can exacerbate depressive symptoms. Incorporating stress-reduction techniques such as deep breathing exercises, progressive muscle relaxation, or yoga can enhance emotional resilience. Setting aside time for hobbies and interests can also serve as a healthy outlet for stress.

5. Social Connections

Maintaining strong social connections is vital for emotional well-being. Engaging with friends, family, or community organizations can provide meaningful support and prevent feelings of loneliness. Making time for social activities, volunteering, or pursuing shared interests can enhance life satisfaction.

Understanding the symptoms of depression, seeking professional guidance, and actively engaging in self- care strategies can empower women to navigate this transitional period with greater confidence and resilience. By embracing a holistic approach that addresses both mind and body, women can foster emotional well-being and improve their overall quality of life during menopause.

Chapter 6: Mental Health Practices for Emotional Well-Being

As hormone levels change and eventually decrease, numerous women encounter symptoms that can impact their mental health, including mood fluctuations, anxiety, depression, and feelings of inadequacy. It is essential to comprehend and address these challenges to ensure emotional well-being during this transitional phase. This chapter will examine various mental health strategies that can assist women in navigating this journey with poise and resilience.

Understanding Menopause and Its Emotional Effects
Menopause generally occurs between the ages of 45 and 55, signifying the conclusion of menstruation and reproductive ability. Although it is often regarded as a natural biological event, the emotional repercussions can be significant. Many women express a wide range of feelings, from relief at the end of menstruation to anxiety regarding aging, identity, and evolving roles within their families and society. Additionally, personal history, cultural context, and life circumstances significantly influence women's experiences during menopause.

Acknowledging these emotional changes is the initial step toward addressing them. Women are encouraged to maintain a journal to monitor their moods, physical symptoms, and triggers. This practice not only enhances mindfulness but also empowers women to take control of their emotional well-being.

Mental Health Strategies for Emotional Well-Being

1. Mindfulness and Meditation
Mindfulness techniques, such as meditation, can be particularly beneficial for managing the emotional turbulence associated with menopause. Meditation promotes a profound connection to the present moment, fostering a sense of tranquility and acceptance. It is advisable to begin with guided sessions lasting five to ten minutes that emphasize breathing techniques. As one becomes more accustomed to the practice, the duration and frequency can be gradually increased.

Moreover, mindfulness can be seamlessly incorporated into daily activities. Simple practices, such as mindful walking or mindful eating, enable women to ground themselves throughout the day, alleviating anxiety and promoting emotional clarity.

2. Cognitive Behavioral Therapy (CBT)
Cognitive Behavioral Therapy (CBT) is an evidence-based therapeutic approach that helps individuals challenge and change unhelpful thoughts and behaviors. Many women find that their self-talk can become negative during menopause, leading to feelings of inadequacy or helplessness. CBT encourages women to identify negative thought patterns, reframe them, and replace them with positive affirmations.

Engaging with a trained CBT therapist can provide support and guidance through this process. Many also find self-help books on CBT techniques useful in developing coping strategies independently.

3. Physical Activity
Regular physical activity has a profound impact on mental

health. Exercise releases endorphins, which are known as "feel-good" hormones, and can alleviate feelings of anxiety and depression. Whether it's brisk walking, yoga, swimming, or cycling, finding a form of exercise that feels enjoyable is key.

Moreover, group activities, such as joining a local dance class or a hiking group, can foster social connections that are crucial for emotional support during menopause.

4. Nutritional Psychology

There is a growing field of research focusing on the connection between nutrition and mental health. During menopause, the body undergoes several changes, and nutrition plays a vital role in managing symptoms and supporting mental well-being. A balanced diet rich in omega-3 fatty acids, antioxidants, and vitamins can positively influence mood and emotional health.

Women are encouraged to incorporate foods like fatty fish, nuts, leafy greens, berries, and whole grains into their diets. Furthermore, practicing mindful eating—being aware of what and how much one is consuming—can enhance the enjoyment of food and support healthy eating habits.

5. Support Networks

Building and nurturing a support network is crucial during menopause. Connecting with friends, family, support groups, or even online communities can provide an outlet for sharing experiences and coping strategies. Many women find relief in talking to others who are undergoing similar challenges, which fosters a sense of belonging and understanding.

Participating in local workshops or seminars focused on menopause can also provide education and community. Such gatherings offer valuable insights into managing symptoms and encourage women to share coping strategies.

6. Professional Help

Sometimes, the emotional challenges of menopause may feel overwhelming and complex. Seeking help from mental health professionals, such as therapists, counselors, or psychologists, can provide a vital source of support. These professionals can offer tailored strategies for dealing with menopause-specific issues, explore underlying concerns, and work collaboratively with individuals to promote emotional resilience.

Cultivating Emotional Resilience

Menopause may present numerous emotional challenges, but it can also be a time of personal growth, transformation, and empowerment. By embracing mental health practices and seeking support, women can navigate this transition with a sense of strength and self-awareness.

Developing emotional resilience involves recognizing the inherent changes and finding ways to adapt. Journaling, engaging in mindful practices, exercising, nurturing relationships, and seeking professional guidance can collectively foster a positive outlook during this crucial phase of life.

Embracing this transition as a natural progression in life, rather than a daunting challenge, can lead to newfound confidence, deeper connections, and a richer understanding of self. The journey through menopause is unique for each woman, but with the right mental health practices, emotional well-being can flourish.

Holistic Approaches to Mental Health

Traditional methods of mental health treatment, which primarily focus on medication and counseling, are increasingly acknowledging the value of integrative therapies that consider the individual as a whole—encompassing mind, body, and spirit. This chapter delves into the principles of holistic mental health approaches, the diverse range of integrative therapies available, and practical routines for emotional wellness that can improve overall mental well-being.

Understanding Holistic Mental Health
Holistic mental health represents a framework that highlights the interconnection of various life dimensions—emotional, social, physical, and spiritual. In contrast to traditional therapies that often treat symptoms in isolation, holistic mental health aims to uncover the root causes of emotional challenges and addresses these through a comprehensive strategy. The underlying belief is that mental well-being transcends the mere absence of mental illness; it embodies a state of equilibrium across multiple facets of life.

Core Principles of Holistic Approaches
Individualization: Each individual's mental health journey is distinct. Holistic approaches are customized to meet the specific needs, preferences, and circumstances of the person. This personalized approach is essential for effective treatment and emotional health.

Whole-Person Perspective: Mental health is intrinsically linked to physical health, interpersonal relationships, and spiritual beliefs. Holistic practices acknowledge that emotional experiences are connected to physical well-being, emphasizing the necessity of nurturing all dimensions of the self.

Prevention and Empowerment: Holistic strategies place a strong emphasis on preventive measures that enable individuals to take control of their mental health. This includes practices designed to foster resilience and enhance emotional intelligence.**Integration of Various Modalities**: Holistic approaches encourage the use of diverse therapeutic tools and practices. Integrating various modalities—such as psychotherapy, mindfulness, nutrition, and physical activities—can enhance overall well-being.

Integrative Therapies for Mental Health

A range of integrative therapies can be incorporated into holistic mental health care. Below are some notable and effective methods:

Mindfulness and Meditation: Mindfulness practices, including meditation, yoga, and breathing techniques, serve as powerful tools for grounding oneself and fostering present-moment awareness. These practices have been shown to reduce stress, enhance mood, and promote emotional regulation.

Nutritional Psychology: The link between diet and mental health is becoming increasingly recognized. Nutritional psychology emphasizes the role of food in mental wellness. A diet rich in fruits, vegetables, whole grains, and healthy fats can improve brain function and emotional stability.

Art and Expressive Therapies: Creative outlets such as art, music, and dance offer profound methods for expressing emotions. These therapies can unlock feelings that may be difficult to articulate verbally and are particularly beneficial for trauma recovery.

Nature Therapy: Spending time in nature, often termed ecotherapy, can play a crucial role in mental health. Nature has a restorative effect, helping to reduce anxiety and improve mood, making outdoor activities an integral part of holistic practices.

Movement and Exercise: Physical activity is not merely beneficial for physical health; it also acts as a natural antidepressant. Regular exercise can alleviate symptoms of anxiety and depression, improve self-esteem, and enhance overall mood.

Acupuncture and Traditional Medicine: Techniques rooted in traditional practices, such as acupuncture and herbal medicine, can supplement modern therapies. These methods often aim to restore balance in the body's energy flows, promoting mental clarity and emotional stability.

Spirituality and Connection: For many, spirituality is a vital aspect of mental health. Engaging in spiritual practices, whether through organized religion or personal spirituality, can provide a sense of purpose, enhance resilience, and promote emotional healing.

Emotional Wellness Routines

Implementing emotional wellness routines can significantly enhance one's mental health. These daily practices foster resilience and emotional regulation while promoting holistic well-being:

Morning Mindfulness Ritual: Start the day with a morning routine that includes meditation, gratitude journaling, or mindful breathing. This sets a positive tone for the day and enhances focus and calmness.

Physical Activity: Integrate movement into daily life, whether through a morning workout, yoga session, or simply a brisk walk. Aim for at least 30 minutes of physical activity most days of the week.

Balanced Nutrition: Plan meals that emphasize whole, nutrient-dense foods and stay hydrated. Being mindful of what we consume can significantly impact our mental states.

Regular Check-ins: Establish a routine for self-reflection. This could involve journaling about feelings, successes, and challenges or utilizing tools to measure mood changes.

Limit Screen Time: Set boundaries around technology use, especially social media, which can adversely impact mental health. Dedicate time each day for digital detox, focusing on connecting with oneself or others in person.

Cultivate Connection: Prioritize meaningful relationships by regularly connecting with loved ones, friends, or community groups. Social support is crucial for emotional resilience.

Bedtime Ritual: Create a calming evening routine that may include reading, gentle stretching, or listening to soothing music. Establishing good sleep hygiene is vital for mental health.

Holistic approaches to mental health provide integrative frameworks for individuals seeking to enhance their emotional wellness. By recognizing the interconnectedness of various life dimensions and incorporating a variety of therapeutic practices, individuals can cultivate resilience, deepen their self-awareness, and improve their overall mental well-being.

Diet and Exercise for Mental Health

Research increasingly highlights the significant influence that diet and physical activity exert on mental health, serving both as preventive strategies and therapeutic approaches. This chapter examines the intricate relationships among nutrition, exercise, and mental well-being, investigating how particular dietary selections and exercise regimens can elevate mood, alleviate anxiety, and enhance cognitive abilities.

The Influence of Nutrition on Mental Health ### Nutritional Psychiatry

Nutritional psychiatry is a growing discipline that investigates the connection between eating patterns and mental health outcomes. Specific nutrients are essential for optimal brain function, neurotransmitter production, and overall psychological well-being.

Essential Fatty Acids: Omega-3 fatty acids, which are abundant in fish, flaxseeds, and walnuts, are vital for maintaining brain health. Studies indicate that these fats may alleviate symptoms of depression and anxiety by enhancing the fluidity of brain cell membranes and supporting neurotransmitter activity.

Vitamins and Minerals: A lack of certain vitamins, especially B vitamins and vitamin D, has been associated with mood disorders. For instance, insufficient folate levels can hinder serotonin synthesis, resulting in depressive symptoms. Consuming foods rich in these nutrients, such as leafy greens, legumes, and fortified cereals, can foster better mental health.

Antioxidants: Oxidative stress is linked to various mental health issues. Diets abundant in antioxidants—found in fruits, vegetables, nuts, and whole grains—can help alleviate this stress and support brain health. For example, berries and broccoli are rich in antioxidants that have been shown to enhance mood and cognitive function.**The Gut-Brain Connection**: Emerging research points to the significance of gut health in mental well-being. The gut microbiome communicates with the brain through the gut-brain axis, influencing mood and behavior. Probiotic-rich foods like yogurt and fermented vegetables are essential for maintaining a healthy gut microbiome, which can correlate with improved mental health and resilience.

Practical Dietary Recommendations

To support mental health through nutrition, individuals can adopt various dietary strategies:

Balanced Diet: A diet rich in whole foods—fruits, vegetables, whole grains, protein sources, and healthy fats—provides the necessary nutrients that promote brain health.

Limit Processed Foods: Highly processed foods, often laden with sugars and unhealthy fats, can exacerbate feelings of anxiety and depression. Reducing these foods while increasing whole foods can create a more favorable diet for mental well-being.

Regular Eating Patterns: Maintaining regular meal times and avoiding excessive skipping of meals can stabilize blood sugar levels and minimize mood swings associated with hunger or blood sugar crashes.

The Power of Physical Activity ### Exercise and Mental Health

Physical activity has long been heralded for its physical health benefits, but its positive impact on mental health is equally significant. Engaging in regular exercise releases endorphins and other neurotransmitters that can lift mood, alleviate stress, and enhance overall psychological well-being.

Reduction of Anxiety and Depression: Exercise has been shown to significantly reduce symptoms of anxiety and depression. A myriad of studies indicates that as little as 30 minutes of moderate exercise several times a week can lead to substantial improvements in mental health.

Stress Relief: Engaging in physical activity can help alleviate stress. The act of moving the body can serve as a powerful distraction, allowing individuals to temporarily escape from negative thoughts and feelings.

Improved Sleep: Exercise can enhance sleep quality, which is critical for mental health. Poor sleep is closely associated with anxiety and depression, and regular physical activity can regulate sleep patterns and improve overall mood.

Boosted Self-Esteem and Cognitive Function: Regular exercise not only enhances physical appearance and fitness levels but also boosts self-esteem and confidence. Additionally, physical activity has been shown to improve cognitive functions such as memory, attention, and processing speed.

Types of Exercise Beneficial for Mental Health

Aerobic Exercise: Activities such as running, cycling, and swimming are particularly effective in producing mood-enhancing effects. Studies have shown that even a brief bout of aerobic exercise can provide immediate mood improvements.

Strength Training: Resistance exercises can also contribute positively to mental health. Research indicates that individuals engaging in regular strength training report fewer symptoms of anxiety and depression.

Mind-Body Practices: Activities that incorporate mindfulness, such as yoga and Tai Chi, are shown to be particularly beneficial for those battling mental health challenges. They not only provide physical health benefits but also enhance emotional regulation and stress resilience.

Creating an Exercise Routine

To reap the mental health benefits of exercise, it is important for individuals to find an activity that they enjoy and can sustain over time. Here are some strategies for establishing a successful exercise routine:

Set Realistic Goals: Start with manageable goals that emphasize consistency rather than intensity. Gradually increase the intensity and duration as confidence and ability grow.

Incorporate Variety: Engage in different forms of

physical activity to prevent boredom and keep motivation high. Mixing aerobic exercises with strength training and recreational activities ensures a comprehensive approach to fitness.

Social Support: Exercising with friends or joining a group can provide motivation and foster social connections, which are beneficial for mental health.

The relationship between what we eat, how we move, and how we feel underscores the importance of adopting healthier lifestyle choices for improved mental health outcomes. Whether through proper nutrition that nourishes the brain or regular exercise that fortifies the body and mind, individuals can empower themselves to cultivate a more resilient and joyful life.

Chapter 7: Emotional Detachment and Reconnection in menopause

In this chapter, we will examine the intricate emotional experiences associated with menopause, the impact of hormonal changes on mood and interpersonal relationships, and the strategies women can employ to navigate this transitional phase, thereby enhancing their connections with themselves and others.

The Emotional Landscape of Menopause
As women transition into perimenopause and ultimately menopause, they may encounter significant emotional fluctuations due to hormonal changes. The decline in estrogen and progesterone levels can affect neurotransmitters in the brain, such as serotonin and norepinephrine, which are crucial for mood regulation. Consequently, women may experience feelings of irritability, anxiety, or depression, which can create emotional distance from partners, friends, and even their own sense of self.

Emotional detachment can present itself in various forms. Some women may feel a sense of numbness or disconnection from their emotions, hindering their ability to engage with their surroundings. Conversely, others may find themselves overly sensitive, overwhelmed by emotions that appear chaotic and challenging to manage. This emotional upheaval can strain relationships, resulting in misunderstandings, conflicts, or a profound sense of isolation.

Understanding Emotional Detachment

Gaining insight into the reasons behind emotional detachment during menopause is essential for addressing the issue. This phenomenon often arises from a blend of physiological changes, societal expectations, and personal life challenges.

The decline in fertility can trigger an identity crisis for many women, leading to feelings of loss, anxiety regarding aging, or concerns about evolving family dynamics as children become independent.

The physical discomforts associated with menopause—such as hot flashes, sleep disturbances, and fatigue—also impact emotional well-being. When physical health declines, emotional health frequently follows suit. Women may retreat inward, not just as a coping mechanism, but also out of a necessity to conserve energy.

Detachment can serve as a protective shield against these intense emotions. It creates a buffer that allows some women to navigate the tumultuous seas of change without becoming overwhelmed by the waves. While this can be beneficial in the short term, prolonged emotional detachment may lead to significant disconnection from loved ones, themselves, and even their passions and interests.

Reconnection: A Journey Back to the Self

Despite these challenges, menopause can also be a time of profound reconnection. If emotional detachment is acknowledged and understood, it presents an opportunity for growth. Women can embark on a journey to reconnect with their emotions and with others, transforming this phase of life into a time of self-discovery and renewal.

Self-Reflection and Awareness: Acknowledging feelings of detachment is the first step toward reconnecting. Journaling can be a powerful tool to process emotions. Writing can help clarify thoughts and feelings, enabling women to address areas of disconnection. Self-reflection can foster an understanding of underlying fears, desires, and needs, allowing for deeper insights into one's emotions.

Creative Expression: Engaging in creative activities can provide an outlet for emotions. Whether through painting, music, or dance, creative expression allows women to channel their feelings in constructive and fulfilling ways. This process often illuminates paths to reconnection with both oneself and others who share similar interests.

Physical Activity and Well-being: Exercise is not only beneficial for physical health but also for emotional well-being. Activities such as yoga, walking, or dancing can boost mood and promote emotional stability. Additionally, a consistent routine of physical activity can serve as a grounding practice, helping to mitigate the emotional swings often associated with menopause.

Seeking Connection with Others: Building and nurturing relationships is essential during this transitional phase. Open communication with partners and friends can clarify feelings and encourage shared experiences. Having candid discussions about the emotional landscape of menopause can foster understanding and strengthen bonds. Participating in support groups or connecting with other women experiencing similar transitions can also provide a sense of community.

Therapeutic Support: For some, seeking the guidance of a therapist or a counselor can facilitate deeper emotional work. Therapy can provide the tools to navigate feelings of detachment and facilitate reconnection, offering strategies to cope with the emotional fallout of menopause.

Embracing the Transition

Menopause is not just an ending; it is also a beginning. Although emotional detachment is a common experience during this time, it can be overcome by fostering a sense of awareness, pursuing self-expression, and reconnecting with oneself and others. This chapter of life can ultimately lead to new perspectives, a deeper understanding of personal identity, and enriched relationships.

The journey through emotional detachment can serve as a catalyst for reconnection, allowing women to emerge into the next phase of life with renewed strength and a more profound sense of self. By embracing both the pains and the joys of this transition, women can transform menopause into an opportunity for growth, intimacy, and new beginnings.

Understanding Emotional Detachment in menopause

Each woman's journey through menopause is distinct; while some may experience relief from prior menstrual challenges, others might encounter emotional detachment and a sense of alienation from themselves and their loved ones. This chapter explores the underlying causes and consequences of emotional detachment during menopause, shedding light on the intricacies of this transformative period.

Hormonal Influences

A significant factor contributing to emotional detachment during menopause is the substantial fluctuation in hormone levels. Estrogen and progesterone are essential in regulating mood and emotional well-being. As women near menopause, the ovaries gradually decrease estrogen production, resulting in fluctuations that can lead to mood swings, anxiety, and depression.

Research indicates that diminished estrogen levels can impact serotonin, a neurotransmitter vital for mood stabilization. As estrogen levels decline, the brain's ability to manage emotions may also diminish, resulting in feelings of disconnection or emotional numbness. For many women, this hormonal shift creates a pervasive emotional fog, hindering their ability to engage with themselves or form meaningful connections with others.

Psychological Factors

Menopause frequently coincides with various life transitions—such as children leaving home, caring for elderly parents, or changes in professional circumstances.

These stressors can exacerbate feelings of emotional detachment, as women grapple not only with their changing bodies but also with their shifting identities.

The psychological ramifications of societal expectations introduce an additional layer of complexity. Women in this phase may feel compelled to project an image of vitality and productivity, leading to an internal struggle between their self-imposed standards and the reality of their emotional experiences. This dissonance can prompt a withdrawal inward, resulting in emotional detachment as they attempt to reconcile their current feelings with their perceived expectations.

The Role of Societal Norms

Cultural narratives surrounding aging and menopause often play a significant role in how women experience this transition. In many societies, there is a stigma attached to aging, and menopause is frequently portrayed negatively, as a time of loss and decline. This cultural framing can lead to feelings of inadequacy and a disconnect from one's previous identity.

Women may internalize these societal beliefs, leading to emotional withdrawal. The absence of open conversations about menopause can exacerbate feelings of isolation, leaving many women to navigate their experiences alone. Emotional detachment can thus become a protective mechanism—an attempt to shield oneself from societal judgment and personal disappointment.

The Physical Manifestations

Physical symptoms such as hot flashes, insomnia, and

fatigue can also contribute to emotional detachment. The discomfort and unpredictability of these symptoms can be overwhelming. Loss of sleep, for instance, may lead to irritability and diminished energy levels, ultimately affecting emotional well-being.

As women attempt to cope with these physical challenges, emotional availability may take a backseat. Relationships may suffer as partners and loved ones notice a shift in engagement. The sense of disconnection, therefore, grows not only from internal struggles but also from the external repercussions that manifest in interpersonal relations.

Effects on Relationships

Emotional detachment can deeply affect relationships, both romantic and familial. Partners may feel frustrated or hurt by their loved one's apparent withdrawal, leading to misunderstandings and a cycle of emotional disconnect. Communication may falter, as the woman grapples with her feelings while struggling to express them effectively.

Adult children may also notice changes, perceiving their mothers as less accessible or engaged. The gap created by this emotional detachment can breed feelings of confusion and resentment on both sides. The emotional disconnect can result in a feedback loop; as relationships suffer, the woman may retreat further into her emotional shell.

Breaking the Cycle: Strategies for Connection

Recognizing and understanding the causes of emotional detachment in menopause is vital for breaking the cycle. Awareness is the first step toward fostering connection, both with oneself and with others. Here are several strategies that women can adopt:

Open Communication: Discussing one's feelings candidly with trusted family members or friends can lessen the burden of isolation. Engaging in dialogue about emotional experiences during menopause fosters understanding and support.

Therapeutic Support: Professional support from a therapist or counselor experienced in menopausal issues can provide a safe space for women to explore their feelings, process changes, and develop coping strategies.

Self-Compassion: Practicing self-kindness is essential. Acknowledging that emotional fluctuations are part of a natural process can provide relief and promote a more positive view of oneself.

Mindfulness and Self-Care: Incorporating mindfulness practices, such as meditation, yoga, or journaling, can help women reconnect with their emotions. Establishing a self-care routine that values emotional well-being as much as physical health is crucial for navigating this transitional period.

Education and Community: Engaging with educational resources about menopause, joining support groups, or participating in community activities can help diminish feelings of alienation and promote a sense of belonging.

By employing strategies to foster awareness and support, women can navigate menopause with grace, embracing both the challenges and opportunities for growth that this unique stage of life presents. The journey through emotional detachment can eventually lead to greater self-understanding and profound connections with others, redefining what it means to thrive during and beyond menopause.

Reconnecting with Yourself in Menopause

This natural stage signifies the end of fertility, but it also heralds an opportunity for profound self-discovery and reconnection. For many, this period brings a variety of emotional, physical, and psychological changes that can be disorienting. Yet, amidst the fluctuations of hormones and life responsibilities, there lies a unique chance to forge a deeper connection with oneself. In this chapter, we will explore practices that encourage self-discovery during menopause and discuss how to build a resilient emotional foundation.

Understanding the Menopausal Transition

Menopause can feel like a tidal wave of change. While some women sail through it with minimal discomfort, others may find themselves grappling with mood swings, anxiety, sleep disturbances, and changes in self-perception. This turmoil can lead to a feeling of disconnect not only with one's body but also with one's identity. Understanding that this stage is natural and that the challenges faced are shared by many is an important first step toward reconnection.

Reflecting on Your Journey

Before embarking on self-discovery practices, it's essential to reflect on your journey up to this point. Consider the following prompts:

What experiences have shaped you in the years leading up to menopause?

How have your roles (whether as a partner, parent,

professional, or caregiver) influenced your sense of self?

What passions or interests have you set aside due to life's demands?

Taking time to journal your responses can help clarify your thoughts and feelings, allowing you to reconnect with aspects of yourself that may have been overshadowed.

Self-Discovery Practices

1. Mindfulness and Meditation

Mindfulness practices can be particularly beneficial during menopause. Engaging in meditation helps quiet the mind and cultivate a sense of presence. Start with just a few minutes each day, focusing on your breath. Allow thoughts to drift in and out without judgment. As you become more comfortable, incorporate visualizations that connect you with your authentic self. Imagine who you want to be in this new phase of life, free from societal pressures and expectations.

2. Creative Expression

Artistic endeavors—painting, writing, dancing, or crafting—can serve as powerful tools for self-exploration. There are no rules in creativity; it's a safe space to express emotions that may be difficult to articulate.

Consider keeping an art journal where you can doodle, write, or vent whatever comes to mind. Hosting a monthly craft night with friends can also foster connection and provide an outlet for shared emotional experiences.

3. Nature and Movement

Physical movement can enhance your mood while providing an opportunity for self-discovery. Whether through yoga, hiking, or dance, find a form of movement that resonates with you. Spending time in nature can be particularly healing; the sights, sounds, and smells can ground your thoughts and reconnect you with your sense of self. Create a ritual around this practice, like taking a weekly walk in a local park, to create consistent moments of mindfulness.

4. Community and Shared Experiences

Connecting with others who are experiencing menopause can alleviate feelings of isolation. Consider forming or joining a support group where you can share stories, challenges, and victories. These shared experiences can create a sense of belonging and remind you that you are not alone in your journey.

Regardless of how you choose to connect—whether in person or virtually—the power of community can foster empathy and understanding, essential elements of emotional resilience.

Building a New Emotional Foundation ### 1. Embracing Change

The key to building a new emotional foundation during menopause lies in embracing change rather than resisting it. Make a conscious effort to shift your mindset—from seeing menopause as an ending, to recognizing it as a beginning. Create affirmations that resonate with you, celebrating your wisdom and strength. Repeat them daily to reinforce your commitment to this new chapter of life.

2. Setting New Goals

Take the time to identify new goals or aspirations that align with your evolving sense of self. These might include career advancements, personal growth projects, or even travel plans. Setting achievable, meaningful objectives can reignite a sense of purpose and motivation, allowing you to reclaim agency in your life.

3. Prioritizing Self-Care

As you embark on this journey of reconnection, prioritize self-care. Make space for activities that nourish your soul—whether it's reading a good book, taking a long bath, or enjoying a hobby you've neglected. By consistently dedicating time to the things that bring you joy, you reinforce the importance of self-love and care in your life.

4. Seeking Professional Support

If emotional turmoil becomes overwhelming or persistent, seeking professional support from a therapist or counselor who specializes in women's health can be incredibly beneficial. A supportive professional can guide you through coping strategies and help navigate the emotional landscape of menopause.

By implementing practices that promote mindfulness, creativity, movement, and community engagement, you can reconnect with your authentic self and build a robust emotional foundation. Embrace this transformative journey with openness and curiosity, and you may find that this new chapter is one of the most rewarding yet.

Chapter 8: Strengthening Relationships During Menopause

This period can serve as a transformative phase, not only for the woman undergoing these changes but also for her interactions with partners, friends, family, and colleagues. As hormonal fluctuations present themselves in both physical and emotional forms, it becomes essential to comprehend and nurture these relationships. In this chapter, we will delve into the complexities associated with menopause and examine strategies for enhancing relationships during this significant stage of life.

Understanding the Impact of Menopause
Menopause generally occurs between the ages of 45 and 55, signifying the conclusion of a woman's reproductive years. It is marked by biological transformations, including a decline in hormone levels, which may lead to symptoms such as hot flashes, sleep disruptions, mood fluctuations, and alterations in libido. These symptoms can influence a woman's self-perception, emotional health, and her interactions with those around her.

Furthermore, societal attitudes towards menopause—often clouded by stigma and misconceptions—can exacerbate a woman's sense of isolation. Some women may feel as though they are losing their identity or confronting an unseen struggle that others fail to comprehend. Conversely, partners may experience feelings of helplessness, confusion, or frustration regarding these changes, particularly if they are unsure how to provide support.

Recognizing menopause as a collective journey rather than an individual experience can greatly improve relational dynamics. Acknowledging shared feelings and experiences cultivates empathy, enhances communication, and ultimately strengthens connections.

Open Communication

A fundamental aspect of fortifying relationships during menopause is the establishment of open communication. Women should be encouraged to express their feelings and experiences related to menopause, while partners should feel comfortable asking questions and voicing their concerns. This exchange can occur in various forms— whether through informal chats, scheduled conversations, or even in therapeutic environments.**Expressing Feelings**: Women should openly share what they are experiencing physically and emotionally. This includes discussing symptoms, mood swings, and how these changes impact their daily life.

Encouraging Questions: Partners should feel comfortable asking questions to better understand what their loved one is going through. This willingness to learn can foster a sense of teamwork.

Setting Boundaries: It's essential for women to communicate their needs and boundaries. For instance, if they need space during a hot flash or feel overwhelmed, having those boundaries respected can lead to less anxiety and more trust.

Building Empathy and Understanding

Empathy is the cornerstone of nurturing relationships during menopause. Partners should actively engage in understanding the emotional and physical turmoil that may accompany this transition. This can involve:

Educating Themselves: Learning about menopause through books, articles, or documentaries can help partners gain insights into what their loved ones are experiencing.

Attending Support Groups: Participation in couples' workshops or support groups can provide valuable perspectives, as individuals hear from others navigating similar challenges.

Validating Emotions: Acknowledging feelings—be it frustration, sadness, or anger—can help women feel heard and understood instead of isolated in their experiences.

Shared Activities and Quality Time

Finding joy amidst the upheaval of menopause is essential for maintaining healthy relationships. Engaging in activities together not only keeps the connection alive but also serves as a reminder of the bond that extends beyond the changes faced. Here are a few ideas:

Physical Activity: Engage in activities like yoga, walking, or cycling. Physical exercise can alleviate some menopausal symptoms and also create a shared goal.

Exploring Interests: Revisit hobbies or create new ones together, whether it's cooking, gardening, or taking workshops. Shared experiences can reignite passion and companionship.

Mindfulness and Meditation: Sometimes the best way to reconnect is through calm and focus. Consider practicing mindfulness or participating in meditation sessions together.

Seeking Professional Help

If the challenges associated with menopause strain relationships significantly, seeking the guidance of a professional may be beneficial. Couples therapy or individual counseling can provide tools and strategies to navigate this transitional period. Professionals can help partners articulate their feelings, teach effective communication strategies, and foster understanding in a safe environment.

Moreover, groups specifically designed for women experiencing menopause can provide a comforting space to discuss shared emotions and experiences. Hearing from others can demystify the process, normalize feelings, and create a support network.

Celebrating Transitions

Menopause signifies the end of one chapter and the beginning of another. It can represent a time of newfound freedom and self-discovery. Celebrating this transition can involve:

Reassessing Goals: This can be a great time for personal growth. Whether it's focusing on career ambitions, health, or travel, setting new goals can provide direction and excitement.

Ritualizing Change: Create rituals that honor this transition period. This could involve a special dinner, a day of pampering, or a weekend getaway that emphasizes the relationship and the new phase of life.

Building a Supportive Community: Strengthening relationships can also mean building a community of friends and peers who understand and support each other's journeys. This camaraderie can alleviate feelings of isolation.

By embracing open communication, empathy, shared activities, and a respectful exploration of emotions, couples can navigate this transition together, emerging with a stronger bond than before. Emphasizing the importance of support, education, and emotional validation ensures that the journey through menopause becomes one of growth, solidarity, and renewed intimacy.

Navigating Emotional Challenges in Relationships

Whether romantic, familial, or platonic, every relationship encounters challenges that can invoke a spectrum of emotions. Navigating these emotional challenges requires effective communication and a deep understanding of one another's needs. This chapter will delve into strategies to foster healthy communication, increase emotional awareness, and cultivate empathy, ultimately leading to stronger, more resilient relationships.

Understanding Emotional Challenges

Emotional challenges in relationships often stem from unmet needs, misunderstandings, or differing expectations. When individuals bring their unique backgrounds, experiences, and emotional histories into a relationship, conflicts can arise. These emotional challenges can manifest as frustration, sadness, anger, anxiety, or even withdrawal. Understanding the root causes of these emotions is essential to facilitating healthy conversations.

The Importance of Emotional Awareness

Emotional awareness is the ability to recognize and understand one's emotions and the emotions of others. It serves as a crucial foundation for effective communication. Individuals who possess emotional awareness can identify their feelings and articulate them more clearly, reducing the likelihood of miscommunication.

Additionally, being attuned to a partner's emotional state fosters empathy and connection. ## Communication Strategies

Effective communication is the cornerstone of navigating emotional challenges in any relationship. Below are several strategies that can enhance communication and help both parties feel heard and understood.

1. Use "I" Statements

One effective way to foster understanding is by utilizing "I" statements rather than "you" statements. For instance, saying "I felt hurt when…" rather than "You always…." shifts the focus from blame to personal feelings. This approach reduces defensiveness and encourages open dialogue, inviting the other person to respond empathetically.

2. Active Listening

Listening is more than simply hearing words; it requires engagement and attention. Active listening involves giving full attention to the speaker, acknowledging their feelings, and reflecting back what they've communicated. This technique not only validates the speaker's emotions but also clarifies any misunderstandings that may arise.

3. Nonverbal Communication

Nonverbal cues—such as body language, eye contact, and tone of voice—play a significant role in communication. Being mindful of nonverbal signals can improve interactions, especially during emotionally charged conversations. Maintaining an open posture and using a calm tone can create a safe space for expressing difficult emotions.

4. Timing Matters

Choosing the right moment for conversation can significantly impact the outcome. Initiating a discussion when both parties are calm and open to dialogue increases the likelihood of productive communication. Avoid discussing sensitive topics during stressful moments or when one person is preoccupied with other concerns.

5. Clarify and Summarize

To ensure mutual understanding, take time to clarify and summarize what has been discussed. This not only reinforces comprehension but also demonstrates that both parties are making an effort to understand each other. Phrases like "What I hear you saying is…" can be particularly effective in confirming understanding.

6. Set Boundaries

Establishing clear boundaries is vital in navigating emotional challenges. Both partners should communicate their limits regarding what is acceptable behavior and what triggers stress or discomfort. Honoring these boundaries fosters respect and safety in the relationship.

Understanding Each Other's Needs

Beyond effective communication lies the importance of acknowledging and fulfilling one another's needs. Each individual has unique emotional requirements, and being proactive in understanding those needs can deepen the connection.

1. Encourage Openness

Creating an environment where both individuals feel safe to express their needs is foundational. Encourage your partner to share their feelings and needs without fear of judgment. Regular check-ins can encourage openness— these can be structured, like weekly conversations about feelings and expectations.

2. Empathy and Validation

Empathy is the cornerstone of understanding. When a partner expresses their feelings, responding with empathy and validation can help bridge the gap between emotional experiences. Validation doesn't necessarily mean agreement; it simply acknowledges the other person's perspective.

3. Recognizing Differences

It's imperative to recognize that individuals may have different needs stemming from diverse backgrounds and life experiences. For example, one partner may prioritize quality time, while another may value acts of service. Identifying these differences can lead to compromises that nurture the relationship.

4. Expressing Needs Clearly

Encouraging each other to articulate needs clearly can eliminate assumptions that often lead to misunderstandings. Use explicit language to express what you require from the relationship. This does not only clarify expectations but also shows a willingness to meet each other halfway.

As partners learn to share their emotions, listen actively, and validate one another, they foster a connection rooted in love, respect, and empathy. Through ongoing practice and dedication, relationships can evolve into resilient bonds capable of weathering the storms of emotional challenges, ultimately leading to deeper intimacy and fulfillment.

Maintaining Strong Relationships in Menopause

The hormonal fluctuations, physical manifestations, and emotional upheaval associated with menopause present distinct challenges for couples. Nevertheless, with appropriate emotional support and effective coping strategies, partners can successfully navigate this transitional period together, thereby enhancing their mutual understanding and connection.

Understanding the Impact of Menopause on Relationships

Menopause frequently brings about various physical symptoms, such as hot flashes, sleep disruptions, and alterations in sexual desire. These symptoms can result in feelings of frustration, irritability, and mood swings, potentially affecting communication and emotional closeness between partners. It is crucial to acknowledge that menopause can introduce stress into a relationship; however, recognizing its possible effects can serve as a foundation for productive discussions.

Communication is Key

While effective communication is essential in any relationship, it becomes particularly important during transitional phases. Partners should foster an open dialogue regarding the changes each individual is experiencing. The person undergoing menopause may feel vulnerable, while their partner might find it challenging to comprehend the physical and emotional impact involved. Creating a safe environment for conversation can promote empathy and minimize misunderstandings.

Suggested Strategies for Improved Communication:
Schedule Regular Check-Ins: Dedicate time to discuss feelings, concerns, and experiences openly. This could be as straightforward as a weekly coffee meeting or an evening stroll.

Practice Active Listening: Acknowledge each other's feelings without interruptions. It is vital for both partners to feel acknowledged and understood.

Use "I" Statements: Rather than assigning blame or making accusations, articulate feelings using "I" statements, such as "I feel overwhelmed" instead of "You don't understand me."## Building Emotional Support Systems

During menopause, individual coping strategies become essential, but couples should also work together to build a supportive environment. Emotional support is multifaceted and can be derived from various sources, including friends, family, and professional help.

Ways to Strengthen Emotional Support Systems:

Encourage External Support: Encourage one another to seek friendships and community support. Engaging in groups geared towards women experiencing menopause, whether in-person or online, can be empowering.

Engage in Mutual Activities: Spend quality time

together doing activities that foster connection, such as cooking, exercising, or participating in hobbies. Shared experiences can reinforce bonds.

Informational Resources: Educate yourselves together about menopause. Books, documentaries, or workshops can shed light on what to expect and how to navigate challenges, which can enhance understanding and empathy.

Couples Therapy as a Resource

While communication and support systems are essential, couples may find great benefit in seeking professional help. Couples therapy can provide a neutral ground for discussing complex feelings and navigating the changes that menopause brings. A trained therapist can help partners communicate more effectively, understand one another's perspectives, and develop tailored strategies for enhancing their relationship.

Benefits of Couples Therapy:

Safe Communication Environment: A therapist can facilitate open dialogue in a non-confrontational setting, helping both partners express their feelings without fear of judgment.

Conflict Resolution: Often, menopause can exacerbate existing conflicts within a relationship. Couples therapy equips partners with skills to address issues constructively.

Personal Growth: Therapy can offer insights into both individual and joint issues that may be impacting the relationship, promoting personal growth and understanding.

Relational Tools: Couples therapists often provide practical tools to improve communication, emotional expression, and mutual support.

Embracing Change Together

Every challenge faced during this transition can serve as a catalyst for enhancing understanding and connection. By fostering open communication, building robust emotional support systems, and considering professional help when necessary, partners can maintain and even strengthen their relationships during this significant life stage.

With the right approach, menopause can be not just a time of challenge but also an opportunity—an opportunity to re-evaluate, reconnect, and rejoice in the enduring bond of partnership. Embracing this journey together can lay the groundwork for a lasting love that withstands the tests of time and transition.

Chapter 9: Communicating Emotional Needs to Loved Ones

Emotional needs encompass our yearnings for love, support, understanding, validation, and intimacy. Acknowledging and expressing these needs can greatly improve our relationships with those we care about. In this chapter, we will examine the significance of articulating emotional needs, explore strategies for effective communication, and discuss potential challenges that may arise in this process.

Understanding Emotional Needs

To communicate our emotional needs effectively, we must first comprehend what they entail. These needs differ among individuals and can be shaped by personal experiences, attachment styles, and previous relationships. Common emotional needs include:
Affection: The necessity for both physical and verbal demonstrations of love and care.
Safety and Security: The wish for emotional stability and reassurance of support.
Appreciation: The desire to feel valued and acknowledged for our identity and contributions.
Understanding: The yearning for empathy and validation of our feelings and experiences.
Autonomy: The need to preserve a sense of self and independence within relationships.
Identifying your own emotional needs is a vital initial step. Take the time to contemplate what you require from your loved ones and how these needs may be reflected in your interactions with them.

The Importance of Communication

Effectively communicating our emotional needs is essential for maintaining a healthy relationship. By expressing our needs clearly, we enable others to understand us more profoundly and cultivate stronger connections. In contrast, neglecting to communicate our needs can result in misunderstandings, resentment, and emotional detachment.### Barriers to Communication

There are various barriers that can hinder effective communication of emotional needs. Fear of vulnerability is a significant one; opening up can feel risky, especially if we have faced rejection or criticism in the past. Cultural background also plays a role; some cultures may discourage the open expression of emotions.

Additionally, misunderstanding or misinterpreting emotional needs can lead to confusion or conflict in relationships.

Strategies for Communicating Emotional Needs

Practice Self-Reflection: Before discussing your emotional needs, take time to explore what they are. Journaling or meditating can help clarify your thoughts and feelings, making it easier to articulate them to others.

Choose the Right Time and Place: Timing is crucial when communicating emotional needs. Select a setting where both you and your loved one feel comfortable—free from distractions—and at a time when neither party is rushed or stressed.

Use "I" Statements: Frame your needs using "I" statements to express your feelings without placing blame. For instance, say "I need more support when I'm feeling down" instead of "You never help me when I'm upset." This approach reduces defensiveness from your partner and encourages open dialogue.

Be Specific: Vague requests can lead to confusion. Be specific about what you need. Instead of saying "I need more affection," consider saying, "I feel loved when you hold my hand or give me compliments."

Be Open to Dialogue: Encourage your loved ones to respond and share their thoughts on your emotional needs. This fosters a nurturing environment where both parties feel valued and understood.

Practice Active Listening: Communication is a two-way street. When your loved one responds, listen actively, noting both their verbal and non-verbal cues. This will help you understand their feelings and needs, cultivating deeper emotional intimacy.

Follow Up: After discussing your emotional needs, check in with each other. This not only reinforces your commitment to each other's emotional well-being but also allows for adjustments as both of you grow and change.

Navigating Challenges

Even with the best strategies, communicating emotional needs can be fraught with challenges. There may be times when your loved one doesn't fully understand your needs or responds in a way that feels dismissive. In such cases, patience is key. It's helpful to approach these moments with compassion, gently reiterating your needs and giving them time to process your feelings.

Similarly, when others express their emotional needs, it's important to listen without judgment, even if their needs are different from yours. This mutual respect fosters a stronger bond, creating a safe space where both parties feel empowered to communicate openly.

Communicating emotional needs is a vital skill that can transform relationships. By understanding our own needs, choosing the right strategies for expression, and being open to dialogue, we can build deeper connections with our loved ones. This chapter has outlined the importance of recognizing and articulating emotional needs, as well as offering practical approaches to enhance communication.

Effective Communication Techniques

For many women, the hormonal fluctuations during this

time can contribute to mood swings, anxiety, and feelings of isolation. Consequently, effective communication becomes vital, allowing women to express their feelings clearly and fostering understanding between them and their loved ones. This chapter explores essential communication techniques that can help navigate the challenges of menopause—highlighting the importance of both expressing feelings and practicing active listening.

The Importance of Clear Expression ### Understanding Your Emotions

Before you can express your feelings to others, it is crucial to understand them yourself. Hormonal changes during menopause can lead to emotional turmoil, including feelings of sadness, irritability, or frustration.

Taking the time to reflect on your emotions can help you articulate them better. Consider keeping a journal to document your feelings. Writing down your thoughts can create clarity and lead to more effective communication when discussing your feelings with others.

Using "I" Statements

One of the most effective ways to communicate your feelings is through the use of "I" statements. This technique involves expressing your feelings and needs without placing blame or triggering defensiveness in the listener. For example, instead of saying, "You never listen to me," reframe it as, "I feel unheard when I try to express my feelings." This approach encourages a constructive dialogue and invites empathy rather than argument.

Choosing the Right Time and Setting

Timing and setting can dramatically influence the

effectiveness of your communication. Choose a calm and private environment where both parties can speak freely without distractions. Discussing sensitive topics during moments of frustration or anger is often counterproductive. Instead, find a moment when both you and your partner or friend are at ease, mentally prepared, and open to conversation.

Active Listening: A Two-Way Street ### What is Active Listening?

Active listening is an essential component of effective communication, especially during emotionally charged situations like those often experienced in menopause. It involves being fully present and engaged in the conversation, demonstrating understanding and empathy towards the speaker.

Techniques for Active Listening

Give Your Full Attention: This means putting away electronic devices, maintaining eye contact, and focusing on the speaker. Show genuine interest in what they are saying.

Reflect and Paraphrase: To ensure understanding, paraphrase what the speaker has said. For example, "What I hear you saying is..." This reiterates that you are listening and valuing their feelings.

Ask Open-Ended Questions: Encourage the speaker to elaborate on their feelings and thoughts. Questions like "How do you feel about that?" or "What can I do to support you?" invite a deeper conversation.

Acknowledge Emotions: Recognizing the speaker's feelings can help create a safe space for open dialogue.

Phrases like "That sounds really tough" or "I can see why you feel that way" validate their experiences and emotions.

Avoiding Interruptions: Show respect by allowing the speaker to finish their thoughts without interruption. This demonstrates that you value their perspective and are genuinely invested in understanding them.

The Role of Empathy in Communication

Empathy is at the heart of effective communication, especially during the transformational period of menopause. By putting yourself in another person's shoes, you can better understand their feelings and reactions. Displaying empathy creates an emotional connection and encourages openness in communication.

Incorporating Empathy into Conversations

Practice Patience: Emotional responses during menopause may not always be rational. Practice patience as you navigate the conversation, reminding yourself that these reactions stem from genuine feelings.

Be Non-Judgmental: Avoid jumping to conclusions or passing judgment on your feelings or those of others. Approach the conversation with compassion and an open mind.

Share Your Own Experiences: If appropriate, sharing your own feelings can help normalize the conversation. However, ensure that the focus remains on the other person's feelings and not shifting the spotlight to yourself.

Navigating the emotional landscape of menopause can be challenging. However, employing effective communication techniques—such as expressing feelings clearly and practicing active listening—can foster deeper understanding and connection between loved ones. These strategies not only help in articulating personal feelings but also create a supportive environment where all parties can share openly.

Building a Supportive Environment

Understanding the social and emotional landscape of menopause is essential for creating a supportive environment that facilitates open dialogue, encourages empathy, and provides practical assistance. This chapter will explore key strategies to cultivate a culture of understanding and support for individuals navigating menopause, outlining actionable steps that can be taken at home, in the workplace, and within the broader community.

Understanding Menopause: The First Step to Support
Educating Yourself and Others

The foundation of a supportive environment begins with education. A lack of knowledge about menopause can lead to misconceptions and stigma. Taking the time to learn about the physiological, emotional, and psychological aspects of menopause is vital for family, friends, and colleagues. Here are some strategies to increase understanding:

Organize Educational Workshops: Invite healthcare professionals to conduct workshops on menopause for employees or community members. This provides a platform for asking questions and dispelling myths.

Distribute Informative Materials: Brochures, online

resources, and books dedicated to menopause can serve as valuable tools for self-education. Sharing these resources in common spaces or within your network can spark conversations about this natural stage of life.

Encourage Open Dialogue: Create opportunities for those affected by menopause to share their experiences. This could be done through support groups or informal discussion circles, fostering a sense of community and belonging.

Promoting Empathy and Compassion

Understanding the biological changes is just one aspect; perhaps more crucial is fostering empathy toward those undergoing the transition. Recognizing that menopause can come with a host of emotional and physical symptoms like hot flashes, mood swings, and sleep disturbances can facilitate compassion. Here are ways to promote empathy:

Active Listening: Encourage individuals to express their feelings and experiences without fear of judgment. Active listening can foster deeper connections and validate the experiences of those going through menopause.

Designate a Safe Space: Create a designated area in homes or workplaces where those experiencing menopause can retreat when in need of support. This area should promote relaxation and comfort, perhaps featuring calming visuals or quiet activities.

Creating Safe Spaces ### In the Workplace

Creating a supportive environment in the workplace is essential, particularly as many women experience menopause while managing their careers. Here are strategies to enhance workplace support:

Flexible Work Arrangements: Implement policies that allow for flexible hours or remote work options, enabling individuals to manage symptoms like fatigue or anxiety without sacrificing productivity.

Menopause Training for Managers: Provide training for managers to help them understand menopause and its impact on employees. This training can reduce stigma and promote supportive interactions.

Comfortable Workspaces: Consider the physical workspace—temperature control is a vital aspect of comfort for those experiencing hot flashes. Allow employees to bring personal fans, adjust thermostats, or take short breaks as needed.

In the Family and Community

A supportive family environment can have profound effects on how one experiences menopause. Here are ideas for creating a nurturing home and community:

Family Education Sessions: Just as in the workplace, educate family members about menopause. This can help spouses and children understand changes in mood or behavior, fostering an atmosphere of patience and support.

Community Networks: Establish community support networks where individuals experiencing menopause can connect for shared experiences and solutions. This encourages bonding and alleviates feelings of isolation.

Incorporate Rituals: Encourage family traditions or rituals focusing on health and wellness. Whether it's cooking nutritious meals together or taking part in relaxation exercises, these rituals can deepen connections and provide necessary support.

Encouraging Open Conversations ### Normalizing Menopause Talks

Creating a culture where menopause can be discussed openly is crucial. Normalizing the conversation can help eliminate stigma:

Use Social Media: Share articles, personal stories, and support group information on social media to raise awareness and normalize discussions around menopause.

Celebrate Milestones: Instead of viewing menopause as a taboo topic, celebrate it as a rite of passage. This could include themed gatherings where experiences are shared, and wisdom is passed down.

Language Matters

Being mindful of language is important when discussing menopause. The words we choose can shape perceptions:

Positive Framing: Use affirming language that emphasizes menopause as a natural phase in life rather than a deficit. Describing it as a "new beginning" can promote a more positive outlook.

Encourage Personal Stories: Sharing personal experiences can humanize the topic and help others feel comfortable expressing their unique journeys. Encourage individuals to share their stories, emphasizing the diversity of menopause experiences.

By educating ourselves and others, designing safe spaces at home and work, and normalizing conversations about menopause, we can create a landscape where individuals feel understood and supported.

Chapter 10: Crying Spells and Emotional Outbursts

The transition into menopause is not merely a physical change; it carries significant psychological ramifications as well. One of the more unexpected elements of this stage in a woman's life is the emotional instability that may arise. In this section, we will examine the factors contributing to episodes of crying and emotional outbursts during menopause, the necessity of recognizing these emotions, and effective methods for managing them.

Comprehending the Emotional Terrain

As women near menopause, generally occurring between the ages of 45 and 55, they experience considerable hormonal shifts. The decline in estrogen and progesterone levels results in not only physical symptoms but also impacts mood and emotional stability. Studies suggest that varying hormone levels can lead to heightened sensitivity, irritability, and an intensified emotional state, which may manifest as crying spells or sudden emotional reactions.

The Influence of Hormones

Estrogen is crucial for the regulation of serotonin, the neurotransmitter associated with feelings of happiness and well-being. A reduction in estrogen can disrupt this equilibrium, rendering women more vulnerable to feelings of sadness or anxiety. Additionally, progesterone has a soothing effect; its decrease can intensify feelings of restlessness. Gaining insight into these relationships aids in understanding why emotional turmoil can be particularly challenging during this period.

Life Changes and Psychological Factors

Menopause often coincides with various life transitions that can amplify emotional responses. For many women, this period includes children leaving home, changes in relationships, and aging parents requiring more care. Each of these transitions can elicit grief, anxiety, and a sense of loss, contributing to the emotional roller coaster experienced during menopause.

Women may also confront their own mortality and reflect on their life achievements, leading to profound feelings of inadequacy or sadness. The culmination of hormonal shifts and life changes creates a perfect storm for emotional instability.

The Experience of Crying Spells

Crying spells can be a surprising occurrence for many women during menopause. They may find themselves tearing up over seemingly trivial matters, whether it's a poignant piece of music, a heartfelt movie scene, or a conversation with a friend. What might have once elicited a mild emotional response can suddenly become overwhelming, and the act of crying may feel uncontrollable.

This phenomenon is not only perfectly normal but can also serve as a vital emotional release. Crying can be therapeutic; it is a way for the body to process and express feelings that might be difficult to articulate.

Acknowledging the legitimacy of these feelings is the first step towards understanding and managing them. ## Normalizing Emotional Outbursts

It is essential to normalize these emotional outbursts during menopause. Society often expects women, especially as they mature, to be composed and emotionally stable. However, menopause shatters this illusion, revealing the depth and complexity of women's emotional lives. By talking openly about these experiences, we can destigmatize them and create a supportive environment for women undergoing this transition.

Open communication with friends, family, and partners can foster understanding and help create a circle of support. Establishing safe spaces to express feelings can empower women to navigate their emotional ups and downs more effectively.

Strategies for Managing Emotional Turmoil

While emotional upheaval during menopause is common, there are various coping strategies women can employ to manage these feelings.

1. **Mindfulness and Relaxation Techniques**

Practicing mindfulness, meditation, and deep-breathing exercises can help ground women during emotional spells. These techniques encourage present-moment awareness and can provide a necessary pause, allowing individuals to process their emotions without becoming overwhelmed.

2. **Physical Activity**

Regular exercise is a potent tool for managing mood swings. Physical activity releases endorphins, which are natural mood lifters. Whether it's a brisk walk, yoga, or dancing, finding an enjoyable form of movement can help mitigate emotional fluctuations.

3. **Healthy Lifestyle Choices**

A balanced diet, adequate sleep, and reduced caffeine and alcohol consumption can make a significant difference in emotional well-being. Nutrients such as omega-3 fatty acids, magnesium, and B vitamins play essential roles in regulating mood.

4. **Social Support Networks**

Engaging with supportive friends, family, or menopause support groups can provide comfort and a sense of community. Sharing experiences with others going through similar challenges can foster camaraderie and reduce feelings of isolation.

5. **Therapeutic Modalities**

Women may benefit from talking to a therapist or counselor specializing in menopause-related issues. Cognitive-behavioral therapy (CBT) can equip women with coping strategies tailored to their specific emotional experiences.

Recognizing these emotional phenomena as normal responses to hormonal changes and life transitions is vital in promoting mental health during this significant life phase. By normalizing these experiences and employing effective coping strategies, women can navigate menopause with resilience and grace, transforming a challenging transition into an opportunity for self-discovery and newfound strength.

Understanding the Root Causes in menopause

As estrogen and progesterone levels undergo fluctuations and ultimately decrease, numerous women encounter a variety of symptoms, with emotional disturbances—often expressed through episodes of crying—being particularly significant. This chapter seeks to thoroughly investigate the underlying causes of these emotional expressions during menopause, examining the biological, psychological, and situational factors that play a role in this aspect of the menopausal journey.

The Biological Landscape

Central to the experience of menopause are hormonal alterations that can disturb the body's natural balance. The reduction of estrogen, in particular, is pivotal. Estrogen is essential not only for reproductive functions but also for influencing various neurotransmitters in the brain, such as serotonin and dopamine, which are vital for mood regulation.

Hormonal Fluctuations

During the transition to menopause, the ovaries decrease their production of estrogen and progesterone, resulting in a range of physical and emotional symptoms. These hormonal changes can lead to mood swings, anxiety, and depression. Research indicates that women who experience significant declines in estrogen may exhibit increased emotional sensitivity, rendering them more prone to crying spells. Therefore, the biological landscape serves as a basis for comprehending the emotional challenges many women encounter during this period.

Neurotransmitter Imbalance

Serotonin, commonly known as the "feel-good" neurotransmitter, is significantly affected by estrogen levels. A decrease in estrogen can result in diminished serotonin production and activity, which may lead to feelings of sadness or hopelessness.

This biochemical connection underscores how physiological changes can elicit intense emotional reactions and crying episodes that many women experience during menopause.

Psychological Dimensions
While the biological aspects are foundational, the psychological context in which menopause occurs also profoundly impacts a woman's emotional state.

Identity and Self-Perception

Menopause often prompts introspection about life's passage, aging, and femininity. The end of reproductive years can trigger a reevaluation of identity and purpose. Women may feel societal pressures to appear youthful and vibrant, leading to feelings of loss and inadequacy. These profound realizations can easily manifest as crying spells, as the emotional release becomes a coping mechanism for grief over lost youth or previously held aspirations.

Life Stressors

The menopausal transition frequently coincides with other life stressors, such as caring for aging parents, changes in career, or the departure of children from the home. This convergence of significant life changes can overwhelm an already susceptible emotional state, leading to increased susceptibility to crying as a means of coping.

The cumulative stress of these experiences can heighten feelings of sadness and frustration, triggering emotional release episodes.

Situational Triggers

It is essential to recognize that certain situational factors can act as triggers for crying spells during menopause.

Social Support and Isolation

Social networks and support systems play a critical role in emotional health during menopause. Those women who experience feelings of isolation or lack adequate social support are often more vulnerable to emotional distress. Conversely, women who have nurturing relationships may experience fewer emotional upheavals, as shared experiences and mutual understanding provide a buffer against emotional turbulence.

Life Events and Transitions

Significant life events—such as the death of a loved one, relationship changes, or retirement—can also trigger emotional release mechanisms. These events can evoke feelings of loss, sadness, or confusion that coincide with the emotional changes seen in menopause. Crying becomes a natural, albeit often misunderstood, response to these stressors.

Coping and Emotional Release Mechanisms

Understanding the root causes of crying spells during menopause allows for better coping strategies to be developed. Emotional release through crying can serve as a crucial outlet for pent-up feelings and lead to momentary relief.

Identifying Triggers

Being aware of specific emotional triggers can empower women to take proactive steps towards emotional regulation. Keeping a journal or practicing mindfulness may help individuals identify patterns and proactively address underlying feelings and reactions to these triggers.

Encouraging Emotional Expression

Encouraging emotional expression is essential in coping with menopausal changes. Crying, rather than being seen as a weakness, can be reframed as a healthy and necessary expression of emotions. Engaging in therapy, support groups, or open discussions with loved ones can provide a safe space for emotional expression, reducing feelings of isolation and enhancing emotional resilience.

Holistic Approaches

Incorporating holistic approaches, such as yoga, meditation, and physical exercise, can also benefit emotional well-being during menopause. These practices not only enhance overall emotional regulation but may also positively influence the biochemical milieu by promoting the release of endorphins and improving serotonin function.

Understanding these root causes provides women with the knowledge to navigate this challenging transition. By addressing and reframing emotional upheavals, while equipping themselves with coping strategies and support, women can find empowerment within their emotional experiences. The journey through menopause can ultimately transform into a period of self-discovery, renewal, and enhanced emotional understanding, leading to a fulfilling new chapter in life.

Managing Sudden Emotional Outbursts

Understanding how to manage intense emotions is essential not only for individual well-being but also for fostering healthy relationships. This chapter seeks to offer immediate coping techniques for handling emotional turmoil and to examine long-term strategies for emotional regulation during this transitional phase.

Understanding Emotional Outbursts in Menopause
Menopause represents a natural biological transition that marks the conclusion of a woman's reproductive years, generally occurring between the ages of 45 and 55. The hormonal changes, particularly the reduction in estrogen levels, can profoundly affect mood and emotional stability. Many women experience heightened irritability, sadness, anxiety, and anger during this period, which can lead to unexpected emotional outbursts.

Recognizing these potential emotional difficulties is the initial step toward effective management. Understanding that these reactions are frequently associated with hormonal shifts can alleviate some of the guilt or shame that may arise. Women should equip themselves with the knowledge and skills necessary to navigate this intricate emotional terrain.

Immediate Coping Strategies
In the event of an emotional outburst, it is vital to have a set of strategies readily available to implement. Here are

some immediate coping techniques:

1. **Pause and Breathe**
When emotions start to escalate, take a brief moment to pause and engage in deep breathing. Deep breathing exercises can help soothe the nervous system and offer a moment of clarity. Inhale deeply through the nose for a count of four, hold for a count of four, and exhale slowly through the mouth for a count of four. Repeat this process until the intensity of your emotions begins to diminish.

2. **Grounding Techniques**

Grounding techniques help anchor you in the present moment and can reduce feelings of anxiety or overwhelm. A simple technique is the "5-4-3-2-1" exercise, where you identify:

5 things you can see,

4 things you can touch,

3 things you can hear,

2 things you can smell, and

1 thing you can taste.

This method helps divert attention from overwhelming feelings and brings awareness to your surroundings. ### 3. **Self-Compassion**

During emotional outbursts, it's easy to fall into self-criticism. Instead, practice self-compassion. Talk to yourself as you would to a friend, expressing understanding and kindness towards your feelings. Remind yourself that it's okay to feel this way during this time of transition.

126

4. **Physical Movement**

Engaging in physical activity can be an effective tool for managing intense emotions. Whether it's a brisk walk, engaging in yoga, or even doing jumping jacks, movement releases endorphins and can significantly improve mood. Sometimes, simply changing your environment can also alleviate intense emotions.

5. **Journaling**

Writing down your feelings can offer a sense of relief and clarity. Set aside a few minutes to express your emotions on paper. This practice can help process feelings, recognize patterns, and illuminate underlying issues contributing to the outbursts.

Long-Term Solutions

While immediate coping strategies are effective for handling sudden emotional outbursts, developing a long-term approach can encourage emotional resilience and stability. Here are some solutions to consider:

1. **Therapy and Counseling**

Engaging with a therapist or counselor can provide the tools and guidance needed to navigate emotional fluctuations during menopause. Cognitive Behavioral Therapy (CBT) in particular can help reframe negative thought patterns and develop healthier responses to emotional triggers.

2. **Mindfulness and Meditation**

Incorporating mindfulness practices, including meditation and yoga, into your daily routine can promote emotional regulation. These practices enhance self-awareness, reduce stress, and cultivate a sense of calm, making it easier to respond to emotional triggers thoughtfully rather than reactively.

3. **Healthy Lifestyle Choices**

Adopting a balanced diet, regular physical exercise, and maintaining a consistent sleep schedule can significantly improve overall emotional stability. Foods rich in omega-3 fatty acids, whole grains, and fruits and vegetables can positively influence mood. Avoiding excessive caffeine and sugar may also help prevent sudden mood swings.

4. **Social Support**

Building a strong network of friends and family who understand what you're going through can provide invaluable emotional support. Engaging in conversations, sharing experiences, or simply spending time with loved ones can foster resilience during challenging moments.

5. **Educate and Prepare**

Educating yourself about menopause and its emotional effects can empower you to anticipate challenges and strategize effectively. Reading literature, attending workshops, or joining support groups can foster a sense of community and shared experience, which can be particularly comforting.

By developing coping skills that can be applied in the heat of emotion and implementing consistent lifestyle adjustments, women can navigate this transitional stage with greater ease, resilience, and confidence.

Chapter 11: The Emotional Rollercoaster of Menopause

For numerous women, menopause represents a profound emotional journey characterized by fluctuations between exhilaration and apprehension, as well as feelings of liberation and grief. This section seeks to examine the emotional dimensions of menopause, highlighting its impact on mental health, interpersonal relationships, and self-perception.

Hormonal Changes: Beyond Physical Manifestations

As women transition into menopause, generally occurring in their late 40s to early 50s, there is a significant decline in estrogen and progesterone levels. This hormonal alteration extends beyond mere physical symptoms; it profoundly influences mood and emotional health. Women may find themselves grappling with heightened irritability, mood fluctuations, anxiety, and even depressive episodes as they navigate this new life stage.

It is crucial to understand that these emotional reactions are not merely responses to physical changes. Rather, they may signify deeper concerns related to personal identity, the aging process, and the various life transitions that frequently accompany menopause. For many, this period coincides with other major life events—such as children leaving home, the responsibility of caring for elderly parents, or nearing retirement—which can intensify feelings of loss, uncertainty, and anxiety.

The Emotional Ups and Downs

The emotional journey during menopause can be compared to an erratic rollercoaster experience. Certain days may evoke a sense of empowerment as women discover a renewed sense of freedom and autonomy. Conversely, other days may be overshadowed by feelings of sadness or a sense of loss.### The Empowering Days

For many, menopause brings an opportunity for self-reinvention. Some women find themselves eager to explore new passions, travel, or focus on hobbies that were previously set aside amid the demands of work and family. This time can present a chance for personal growth, encouraging women to prioritize their own needs and desires. This shift can create a feeling of liberation, as they no longer navigate monthly cycles or the burdens of contraception.

The Overwhelming Days

Conversely, the emotional toll of menopause can be significant. Fluctuating hormones can lead to unexpected tears, frustration with minor inconveniences, or feelings of melancholy. Women may find themselves questioning their self-worth or aging process, grappling with fears of invisibility, or feeling disconnected from their younger selves. This sense of loss, combined with the invasive nature of menopausal symptoms, can create feelings of overwhelm and despair.

Navigating Relationships During Menopause

The emotional rollercoaster of menopause does not occur in isolation. Its impact often reverberates through relationships, both personal and professional. Partners may struggle to understand the changes occurring in their spouse, creating potential tension and misunderstanding. Open and honest communication is essential, as partners can support each other through this transition.

Moreover, friendships can play a vital role in navigating the emotional ups and downs of menopause. Sharing experiences with other women can foster connection and provide a support network that alleviates feelings of isolation. Support groups, whether in person or online, can help women realize that they are not alone in their struggles and victories.

Addressing Emotional Health: Tools and Strategies

While the emotional journey of menopause can be challenging, there are tools and strategies that can help women manage their mental well-being:

Mindfulness and Relaxation Techniques: Practices such as meditation, yoga, and deep-breathing exercises can help reduce anxiety and promote emotional stability. These techniques foster a greater awareness of emotional shifts, helping women develop coping mechanisms.

Physical Activity: Regular exercise has been shown to improve mood and reduce anxiety. Whether through walking, dancing, or more structured workouts, physical activity can help mitigate some of the emotional challenges of menopause.

Seeking Professional Help: Therapy or counseling can be beneficial for women experiencing significant emotional distress. A mental health professional can provide coping strategies and a safe space to express feelings.

Healthy Lifestyle Choices: A balanced diet, proper hydration, and ample sleep can positively influence emotional health during menopause. Reducing caffeine and sugar intake, for instance, can help regulate mood swings.

Building a Support Network: Connecting with friends, family, or support groups can provide comfort and understanding. Sharing experiences and listening to others can create a sense of belonging and reduce feelings of isolation.

Embracing the Journey

Ultimately, menopause is a transition that marks the end of one chapter and the beginning of another. While the emotional rollercoaster can be daunting and filled with uncertainties, it can also be an opportunity for renewal and self-discovery. By acknowledging the complexities of the emotional landscape and using effective strategies for support, women can navigate this phase with resilience and grace.

What Causes the Emotional Rollercoaster?

It's a familiar experience for many, marked by extreme highs and lows that can leave us feeling exhilarated one moment and utterly drained the next. But what underpins these dramatic shifts in emotions? In this chapter, we will delve into two primary factors contributing to this emotional turbulence: hormonal fluctuations and external stressors.

Hormonal Fluctuations: The Body's Internal Compass

Our emotions are deeply intertwined with our biology, and one of the most significant influences on our mood resides in the realm of hormones. Hormones are biochemical messengers that facilitate communication within our bodies, influencing everything from growth and metabolism to mood and emotional stability.

Their fluctuations can be attributed to various factors including age, sex, and even the time of day. ### The Role of Key Hormones

Estrogen and Progesterone: In women, the menstrual cycle exemplifies how hormonal fluctuations can trigger emotional ups and downs. During the luteal phase, when progesterone levels peak, many women report feelings of irritability and mood swings, commonly associated with Premenstrual Syndrome (PMS). The dramatic drop in estrogen and progesterone just before menstruation can also lead to feelings of melancholy or anxiety.

Testosterone: In men, testosterone plays a critical role too. While often linked to aggression, low levels can lead to fatigue, depression, and a decline in emotional regulation, resulting in moodiness and irritability.

Cortisol: Often termed the "stress hormone," cortisol is produced by the adrenal glands and plays an essential role in the body's stress response. Chronic stress can lead to sustained high levels of cortisol, which not only affects the physical body but can also provoke anxiety, depression, and emotional instability.

Serotonin: Known as the "feel-good" hormone, serotonin is crucial in regulating mood, anxiety, and overall emotional well-being. Low serotonin levels can result in feelings of sadness, irritability, and even cause conditions such as depression.

The interplay of these hormones and others means that our emotional state can shift dramatically based on biological changes alone, illustrating why understanding our bodies is pivotal in managing emotional well- being.

External Stressors: The Environment We Navigate

While hormonal fluctuations are pivotal in shaping our emotions, they do not operate in isolation. Our emotional landscape is also molded by external influences — the world around us often acts as a catalyst for our feelings, igniting or amplifying our emotional responses.

The Impact of Daily Stressors

Work-Related Stress: Occupational demands can introduce significant external pressure, whether from looming deadlines, workplace conflicts, or a lack of support. This stress can greatly impact mental health, leading to burnout, anxiety, and mood instability.

Personal Relationships: Our interactions with family, friends, and romantic partners can either nurture or frustrate us. Conflicts, misunderstandings, or the burden of expectations can lead to emotional distress, while supportive relationships can help buffer against the rigors of life.

Societal Expectations: External societal pressures, including the pursuit of success, perfectionism, and the need for social acceptance, can create chronic stress that affects our emotional health. Fears of judgment or failure can exacerbate feelings of inadequacy and anxiety.

Global Events: The pervasive impact of global issues, such as economic instability, political unrest, or health crises (as seen during the COVID-19 pandemic), can heighten feelings of uncertainty and fear, contributing to an emotional rollercoaster for many.

The Interplay of Internal and External Influences

It's crucial to recognize that hormonal fluctuations and external stressors often interact, amplifying emotional responses. For instance, a woman experiencing PMS may find that stress from her job exacerbates her irritability. Alternatively, a man under stress from a relationship may experience elevated cortisol levels, further complicating his ability to manage his emotions.

Understanding this reciprocal relationship between internal biology and external circumstances is essential for managing emotional well-being. It emphasizes the need for a holistic approach to mental health, one that accounts for both the physiological and situational factors contributing to emotional fluctuations.

Strategies for Navigating the Emotional Rollercoaster

Armed with the understanding of what drives our emotional ups and downs, we can cultivate strategies to navigate this turbulent terrain better:

Mindfulness and Meditation: Practicing mindfulness helps create a buffer against stress, allowing individuals to respond rather than react emotionally.

Exercise: Physical activity can lead to the release of endorphins, the body's natural mood lifters, while also helping to regulate hormonal imbalances.

Open Communication: Engaging in dialogue about feelings can help alleviate emotional burdens and forge stronger connections with others, offering support when needed most.

Professional Support: Seeking guidance from mental health professionals can provide tools to manage emotional fluctuations effectively, offering strategies tailored to individual circumstances.

Healthy Lifestyle Choices: A balanced diet, adequate sleep, and reducing caffeine and sugar intake can assist in regulating mood and hormonal balance.

By recognizing and understanding these influences, we can take proactive steps to manage our emotions more effectively, creating a smoother ride through the inevitable highs and lows of life. Embracing a multifaceted approach enables not just survival but a flourishing existence amid life's unpredictability.

Balancing Mood Swings

Understanding and addressing these mood fluctuations is crucial for maintaining overall well-being during this transition. This chapter delves into effective emotional regulation techniques, emphasizing the role of mindfulness and meditation in fostering emotional resilience.

Understanding Mood Swings in Menopause

The onset of menopause signifies the end of a woman's reproductive years, typically occurring between the ages of 45 and 55. During this phase, fluctuations in estrogen and progesterone levels can lead to various physiological and psychological symptoms. Mood swings may manifest as sudden feelings of anger, unexpected sadness, or periods of inexplicable joy. Recognizing that these emotional responses are tied to hormonal changes can provide an important context for coping strategies.

The Impact of Hormonal Changes

Hormones play a significant role in regulating mood. Estrogen, for example, influences neurotransmitters such as serotonin and dopamine, which are critical for mood stabilization. As levels of these hormones decline, it can result in a more reactive emotional state. Understanding this connection can help women frame their experiences during menopause, allowing them to approach their mood swings with greater compassion and less frustration.

Emotional Regulation Techniques

Emotional regulation involves strategies to manage and respond to emotional experiences effectively. When it comes to mood swings during menopause, several techniques can be beneficial:

1. **Cognitive Behavioral Techniques**

Cognitive Behavioral Therapy (CBT) techniques can help in reframing negative thoughts. By identifying cognitive distortions—such as catastrophizing or all-or-nothing thinking—women can learn to challenge and replace these thoughts with more balanced, realistic ones. Keeping a thought diary can be a powerful tool for recognizing patterns and triggering events related to mood changes.

2. **Journaling**

Writing about one's thoughts and feelings can provide an outlet for emotional expression. Journaling allows for reflection on mood changes, helping women to identify triggers and develop healthier coping strategies. By making these emotions tangible, it is easier to process and manage them.

3. **Physical Activity**

Regular physical activity is known to boost endorphins—

the body's natural mood elevators. Engaging in activities such as walking, yoga, or dancing can significantly enhance mood and provide a sense of achievement and control.

4. **Social Support**

Connecting with friends, family, or support groups can provide an emotional safety net. Sharing experiences with others who understand the challenges of menopause can foster feelings of validation and support, reducing the sense of isolation that often accompanies this life stage.

Mindfulness and Meditation: Grounding Techniques

Incorporating mindfulness and meditation practices can further aid in managing mood swings during menopause. These techniques promote emotional awareness and help cultivate a more resilient response to distress.

1. **Mindfulness Practices**

Mindfulness involves being fully present in the moment, acknowledging thoughts and emotions without judgment. Practicing mindfulness can help women recognize mood fluctuations as temporary states rather than permanent feelings. This awareness creates space for understanding and responding to emotions constructively.

How to Practice Mindfulness:

Body Scan Meditation: Lay or sit comfortably and bring awareness to different body parts, noticing sensations without judgment.

Breathing Exercises: Focus on the breath, observing inhalation and exhalation. Use deep, slow breaths to promote calm.

2. **Guided Meditation**

Guided meditation, often available through apps or online resources, can provide a structured way to engage with meditation. These sessions can focus on themes such as stress reduction, emotional healing, and self- compassion, directly addressing the emotional upheaval many experience during menopause.

3. **Gratitude Journaling**

Incorporating gratitude into mindfulness practices can also uplift mood. By regularly writing down things one is grateful for, women can shift their focus towards positive aspects of life, creating a buffer against negative emotions.

Building a Daily Mindfulness Routine

To effectively manage mood swings, establishing a daily mindfulness routine can be invaluable. Here is a simple framework to follow:

Morning Mindfulness: Begin each day with a few minutes of quiet reflection or meditation. Setting intentions for the day can help frame emotional responses.

Mindful Breaks: Throughout the day, take short breaks to practice mindfulness. This could involve a few minutes of focused breathing or stepping outside to appreciate nature.

Evening Reflection: At the end of the day, reflect on what went well and what emotions were experienced. Journaling or simply contemplating these moments can enhance emotional awareness.

Consistent Practice: Like any skill, mindfulness takes

practice. Establishing a routine can help cultivate resilience, making it easier to navigate emotional ups and downs.

Mindfulness and meditation not only foster emotional resilience but also cultivate a deeper understanding of one's experiences. By integrating these practices into daily life, women can embrace this transition with greater grace, ultimately leading to a more balanced emotional landscape during menopause. Mindful awareness and self-compassion become invaluable allies in this journey, transforming challenges into opportunities for personal growth and insight.

Chapter 12: Managing Increased Anger and Frustration

This chapter will examine the fundamental reasons behind the emotional experiences during menopause, their effects on everyday life, and practical approaches for managing these feelings.

Understanding the Emotional Rollercoaster

The Physiological Basis
To comprehend the emotional upheavals associated with menopause, it is essential to recognize the physiological changes involved. Menopause generally occurs between the ages of 45 and 55, signifying the conclusion of a woman's reproductive phase as levels of estrogen and progesterone decline. These hormonal shifts can significantly influence mood regulation, resulting in reduced serotonin levels and increased irritability and anger.

The resulting hormonal imbalance may initiate a series of physical symptoms, including hot flashes, sleep disruptions, and fatigue, which can further amplify feelings of frustration. When these symptoms are compounded by societal expectations, personal demands, and life transitions—such as caregiving roles or changes in identity—it is understandable that many women experience overwhelming emotions.

The Psychological Impact
In addition, the psychological dimensions of entering menopause warrant attention. This transition often brings

forth insecurities related to aging, alterations in physical appearance, and changes in interpersonal relationships. Such issues can heighten feelings of frustration and anger, leading to a profound sense of loss or grief regarding life changes. Furthermore, the accumulated stress from various life responsibilities, including career challenges, family dynamics, and personal goals, can exacerbate these emotional responses.

Recognizing Triggers

Understanding personal triggers is key to managing anger and frustration during this phase. Reflect on situations or interactions that prompt these feelings. Common triggers include:

Physical Discomfort: Hot flashes, night sweats, and fatigue can increase irritability and reduce patience.

Life Transition: Changes in family dynamics, such as children leaving home or increased responsibilities as a caregiver for aging parents, can create feelings of overwhelm.

Social Isolation: Feeling disconnected from friends or support networks can lead to an increase in negative emotions.

Work Stress: Balancing career demands with personal life can intensify feelings of anger, particularly in high-stress environments.

Self-Image Issues: Changes in body image and self-perception can lead to frustration, particularly if these changes are not accepted.

Strategies for Management

While it can be challenging to navigate heightened emotions during menopause, there are numerous strategies that can help women regain control and foster emotional well-being.

1. Mindfulness and Meditation

Practicing mindfulness and meditation can significantly reduce feelings of anger and frustration. Taking time to pause, breathe deeply, and focus on the present moment can help cultivate a sense of calm. Guided meditations specifically designed for emotional regulation may be particularly beneficial.

2. Physical Activity

Regular exercise is a powerful tool for managing mood. Physical activity stimulates the production of endorphins, which can enhance mood and reduce feelings of irritability. Whether it's a daily walk, yoga, dancing, or any form of movement, finding an enjoyable way to stay active can help mitigate emotional turbulence.

3. Nutrition

A balanced diet can have a profound impact on mood. Foods rich in omega-3 fatty acids, such as fatty fish, flaxseeds, and walnuts, can help stabilize mood. Likewise, incorporating fruits, vegetables, whole grains, and lean proteins provides the body with essential nutrients that may alleviate emotional fluctuations.

4. Build a Support Network

Establishing a support network of friends, family, or support groups can alleviate feelings of isolation. Sharing experiences and feelings with others who are navigating similar changes can provide comfort and validation. Don't hesitate to reach out to loved ones or consider therapy if needed.

5. Expressive Outlets

Finding healthy outlets for expressing anger is crucial. Journaling, art, or even talking to a trusted friend can help release pent-up feelings. Engaging in hobbies or activities that bring joy can also shift focus away from frustration.

6. Seek Professional Help

If feelings of anger and frustration become unmanageable, seeking professional help from a therapist or counselor can provide additional support. Cognitive-behavioral therapy (CBT), for instance, can help individuals identify patterns of thought and behavior that contribute to emotional distress and develop coping strategies.

By recognizing personal triggers and implementing effective strategies, women can navigate this challenging transition with greater ease. Remember, menopause is not just an end, but also a beginning—a chance to embrace a new chapter in life with understanding, resilience, and empowerment.

Causes of Menopause-Related Anger

The transition into menopause can represent liberation from menstruation and the opportunity to embrace new phases of life; however, it is frequently accompanied by a complex set of emotional and physical challenges. Among these challenges, mood fluctuations and feelings of anger may arise, resulting in considerable distress. To comprehend the origins of menopause-related anger, it is crucial to examine both the psychological aspects and the physical discomforts that contribute to this emotional upheaval.

1. Hormonal Changes
Central to menopause is a notable alteration in hormone levels, particularly estrogen and progesterone. These hormones are vital not only for reproductive health but also for mood regulation. As estrogen levels decline during menopause, women may encounter various emotional disturbances, including increased irritability and anger. The brain's sensitivity to hormonal variations means that these fluctuations can influence neurotransmitters such as serotonin and dopamine, which are essential for mood stability. A reduction in these neurotransmitters may lead to heightened sensitivity to stressors, making women more susceptible to feelings of anger and frustration during this transitional phase.

2. Cognitive and Emotional Shifts
Menopause is often associated with a range of cognitive and emotional shifts. Women may experience "brain fog," which manifests as difficulties in concentration and memory.

This confusion or forgetfulness, linked to cognitive decline, can result in frustration and expressions of anger. Hormonal changes directly impact cognitive appraisal— the manner in which individuals perceive and interpret situations—potentially distorting perspectives and responses.

This misinterpretation, combined with emotional reactions, can create a cycle of escalating anger.Additionally, emotional changes, including increased anxiety and depression, can exacerbate feelings of anger. Women may feel overwhelmed by the sense of loss associated with aging or the transition from one life stage to another. This grief can manifest as anger, directed either inward towards oneself or outward toward others.

3. Physical Discomforts

The physical symptoms of menopause, including hot flashes, night sweats, and sleep disturbances, play a significant role in generating feelings of irritability and anger. Hot flashes can be disruptive and humiliating, leading to heightened feelings of anxiety or embarrassment. The constant battle with these uncomfortable physical symptoms can create a wearisome emotional landscape.

Furthermore, sleep disturbances impact mood significantly. The inability to achieve restorative sleep due to night sweats or anxieties associated with this life transition can lead to chronic fatigue. Sleep deprivation has been linked to increased irritability and emotional reactivity, making it more difficult to cope with everyday stressors, and can trigger episodes of anger that seem disproportionate to the specific triggers.

4. Societal and Relationship Changes

The menopausal transition often coincides with significant life changes, such as shifts in family dynamics, aging parents, or transitioning children. These adjustments can create additional stress, leading to feelings of anger as women navigate their roles within their families and society. For many, the feeling of being unsettled during this time can contribute to a sense of being unmoored, leading to spontaneous anger outbursts.

Moreover, societal attitudes toward aging women can contribute to feelings of inadequacy and frustration. Women may feel dismissed or stereotyped in the workplace or in social settings as they age, which can trigger feelings of anger about their treatment. The internalization of societal expectations and norms regarding femininity and aging can create a potent mix of emotions that surface as anger.

5. Coping Strategies and Support Systems

Understanding the multifaceted nature of menopause-related anger is crucial for developing effective coping strategies. Women can benefit from both psychological and physical support systems during this transition. Engaging in stress-reduction techniques such as mindfulness, yoga, and exercise can mitigate the emotional and physical symptoms of menopause.

Building a supportive network, whether through friendships, support groups, or counseling, can provide an outlet for expressing frustrations and sharing experiences. Empowering women through education about menopause and its effects can also foster resilience, encouraging proactive management of the associated emotional challenges.

The experience of anger during menopause is a complex interplay of hormonal, psychological, and physical factors, intertwined with societal influences and personal life changes.

Transforming Anger into Calmness

The hormonal changes that occur during this period can lead to heightened emotions such as anger, frustration, and irritability. While these feelings can be distressing, the ability to convert anger into tranquility presents a significant opportunity for developing emotional resilience and overall well-being. This chapter delves into strategies for managing anger and calming techniques that can assist women in gracefully navigating this transitional phase.

Understanding Anger in Menopause

To effectively address anger during menopause, it is crucial to comprehend its origins. Fluctuations in hormones, particularly the reduction of estrogen and progesterone, can influence neurotransmitters and brain chemistry, resulting in mood swings and heightened irritability. Furthermore, life transitions—such as aging, changes in relationships, and career shifts—can intensify these emotional responses. Recognizing that these feelings are a natural aspect of the menopausal journey is the initial step toward transforming them.

The Role of Anger
Anger frequently acts as an emotional reaction to unmet

needs or perceived threats. In the context of menopause, this anger may arise from feelings of loss of control, societal pressures, or personal insecurities. It is essential to acknowledge anger as a legitimate emotion that can reveal underlying concerns. Rather than suppressing this anger, we can approach it with empathy and curiosity, allowing us to explore the deeper issues involved.## Anger Management Strategies

Now that we have a clearer understanding of anger, let's explore practical strategies for managing it effectively during menopause.

1. **Identify Triggers**

Keep a journal and record instances of anger that arise. Note the circumstances, feelings, and physical sensations that accompany these emotions. Identifying patterns in your triggers can help you anticipate and manage reactions more effectively in the future.

2. **Practice Mindfulness and Self-Awareness**

Mindfulness allows us to become aware of our emotions without judgment. Simple techniques such as deep breathing, progressive muscle relaxation, or focused meditation can help center your thoughts. For instance, taking a few moments to breathe deeply when you feel anger rising can help create space and clarity before reacting.

3. **Communicate Openly**

When anger arises, it is crucial to communicate feelings in a constructive manner. Use "I" statements to express your feelings without blaming others. For example, "I feel overwhelmed when I have too many tasks to juggle" is more effective than "You never help around the house." Open dialogues foster understanding, reducing feelings of isolation and frustration.

4. **Set Boundaries**

Sometimes, anger stems from feeling overwhelmed by expectations—be it from family, work, or society. Setting clear boundaries around your time and energy can significantly reduce feelings of resentment and anger. Learn to say no when necessary; prioritizing your mental health is vital.

5. **Seek Support**

Share your experiences with trusted friends or family members who understand what you're going through. Consider joining support groups specifically for women in menopause. Bonding over shared experiences can alleviate feelings of isolation and offer valuable perspectives.

Calming Practices

In addition to anger management strategies, incorporating calming practices into daily routines can enhance emotional regulation and foster a sense of peace.

1. **Physical Activity**

Regular exercise releases endorphins, which naturally improve mood and reduce stress. Engage in activities you enjoy, whether it's yoga, dancing, swimming, or simply taking a walk in nature. Physical movement is not only a distraction from anger but also a valuable outlet for pent-up energy.

2. **Explore Creative Outlets**

Expressing anger creatively can be incredibly therapeutic.

Try journaling, painting, or playing music as a way to channel those intense feelings into something productive and healing. Reflecting on emotions through creative processes can provide clarity and facilitate emotional release.

3. **Cultivate Relaxation Techniques**

Incorporate relaxation techniques into your daily routine. Consider practices such as tai chi, guided meditation, or aromatherapy with calming scents like lavender and chamomile. These techniques can deepen relaxation, helping counteract intense emotions and bring about mental stillness.

4. **Establish a Self-Care Routine**

Prioritize self-care as a fundamental aspect of managing anger and stress. Schedule time for activities that nourish your body and soul—whether that's reading a book, taking a warm bath, or enjoying time in nature. Self-care is a proactive way to fill your emotional reserves, making it easier to respond calmly to difficult situations.

5. **Practice Gratitude**

One of the most powerful ways to shift focus from anger to calmness is to cultivate a gratitude practice. Each evening, write down three things for which you are grateful. This simple act can help foster a positive mindset and diminish feelings of frustration by drawing attention to the good in your life.

By adopting effective anger management strategies and calming practices, women can transform volatile emotions into pathways for understanding and personal empowerment.

Conclusion

As we conclude our exploration of emotional stability during menopause, it is essential to recognize that this transformative phase of life is not a journey to be faced alone. The emotional fluctuations, challenges, and growth that come with menopause are shared experiences among many women. Understanding that you are not alone can be a comforting and empowering realization.

Throughout this book, we have delved into the biological, psychological, and social aspects of menopause, shedding light on the emotional turmoil some women may face. We have discussed practical strategies, tools, and techniques to foster emotional stability during this time, ranging from mindfulness practices and physical health considerations to the importance of social support and professional guidance.

Remember, emotional stability is not about suppressing feelings or striving for constant happiness; instead, it's about acknowledging your emotions, understanding their origins, and equipping yourself with the means to navigate through them with grace and resilience. Embracing mindfulness can help ground you and promote self-compassion during moments of difficulty.

Minimizing feelings of isolation can be equally transformative. Reach out to friends, family members, or support groups who can provide a listening ear, share experiences, and offer encouragement. Don't hesitate to seek professional help if you find that your emotional well-being is significantly impacted; mental health professionals can provide valuable resources and coping strategies tailored to your unique circumstances.

As you move forward, remember that this time of life, while fraught with challenges, is also an opportunity for growth, self-discovery, and empowerment. Every woman's journey through menopause is unique, but within its shared challenges lie countless possibilities for resilience and renewal.

May you embrace this season of change with compassion for yourself and a commitment to nurturing your emotional health. You have the inner strength to navigate this transition, and by prioritizing emotional stability, you are setting the foundation for a vibrant and fulfilling life on the other side of menopause.

Thank you for joining us on this journey to emotional stability. We wish you all the best as you move forward into this new chapter of your life. Embrace it with courage, and remember—the best is yet to come.

Biography

Hillary Palms is a distinguished expert in the realm of personal wellness and emotional management, with a special focus on the transformative journey of menopause. With a deep-seated passion for helping individuals navigate the intricate landscape of hormonal changes and stress management, Hillary has dedicated her career to empowering others to embrace their inner strength and achieve a balanced, fulfilling life.

A graduate of renowned health and wellness programs, Hillary has amassed a wealth of knowledge through years of study and hands-on experience. Her expertise is not just academic; it's deeply personal. Having faced her own challenges with menopause and the emotional rollercoaster it brings, Hillary combines scientific insight with genuine empathy, offering readers a uniquely relatable perspective.

In her groundbreaking book, Hillary delves into the world of Palms, weaving together practical advice, personal anecdotes, and cutting-edge research. Her goal is simple yet profound: to provide readers with the tools they need to manage their symptoms, reduce stress, and reclaim their vitality. Hillary's engaging writing style and persuasive tone make complex concepts easy to understand, inspiring readers to take proactive steps towards their well-being.

Beyond her professional pursuits, Hillary is an avid gardener and a lover of the great outdoors. She finds solace in nature, which she believes plays a crucial role in maintaining emotional balance and overall health. Whether she's tending to her lush garden or hiking through scenic trails, Hillary embodies the principles of holistic wellness she so passionately advocates.

Join Hillary Palms on a transformative journey towards better health and emotional resilience. With her guidance, you'll discover the power within to navigate life's changes with grace and confidence.

Glossary: Emotional Stability During

Menopause

1. **Menopause**

The natural cessation of menstruation experienced by women, typically occurring between the ages of 45 and 55. This period is marked by significant hormonal changes, particularly the decline of estrogen and progesterone, which can lead to various physical and emotional symptoms.

2. **Perimenopause**

The transitional period leading up to menopause, often starting in a woman's 30s or 40s. During perimenopause, hormonal fluctuations can lead to irregular menstrual cycles and a variety of emotional changes, such as mood swings and increased anxiety.

3. **Hormonal Fluctuations**

Variations in hormone levels, particularly estrogen and progesterone, that occur during menopause and perimenopause. These fluctuations can contribute to emotional instability, irritability, and depression in some women.

4. **Hot Flashes**

A common symptom of menopause characterized by sudden feelings of warmth, often accompanied by sweating and rapid heartbeat. Hot flashes can disrupt sleep and contribute to mood disorders, thereby affecting emotional stability.

5. **Sleep Disturbances**

Changes in sleep patterns that may occur due to hormonal

shifts during menopause. Insomnia or frequent waking can exacerbate feelings of anxiety or irritability, negatively impacting emotional well-being.

6. **Mood Swings**

Rapid and intense fluctuations in mood that can occur due to hormonal changes. Women may find themselves feeling happy one moment and irritable or sad the next, which can make emotional stability challenging.

7. **Anxiety**

A feeling of worry, nervousness, or unease that can become heightened during menopause due to hormonal changes. This emotional state can interfere with daily life and well-being.

8. **Depression**

A common mental health condition characterized by persistent feelings of sadness and loss of interest. Menopausal women may experience increased risk of depression due to hormonal changes, sleep disturbances, and life stressors.

9. **Coping Mechanisms**

Strategies and techniques that individuals use to manage stress, emotions, and challenges. Effective coping mechanisms can enhance emotional stability during menopause and may include mindfulness, therapy, and exercise.

10. **Mindfulness**

A mental practice that involves staying present and fully engaging with the current moment. Mindfulness practices, such as meditation or deep breathing exercises, can help women cultivate emotional balance during menopause.

11. **Support Systems**

Networks of family, friends, or professionals that provide emotional and practical support. Strong support systems can play a crucial role in helping women navigate the emotional challenges of menopause.

12. **Hormone Replacement Therapy (HRT)**

A medical treatment that involves taking hormones to alleviate symptoms associated with menopause. For some women, HRT may improve not only physical symptoms but also enhance emotional stability.

13. **Lifestyle Modifications**

Adjustments to daily habits and routines that promote physical and emotional health. These may include regular exercise, a balanced diet, and adequate sleep—all of which can foster emotional stability during menopause.

14. **Psychoeducation**

The process of providing information and education about mental health issues and emotions, helping individuals understand their experiences during menopause. This knowledge can empower women to seek help and implement strategies for improving emotional well-being.

15. **Therapeutic Interventions**

Various treatment methods designed to address emotional challenges, including cognitive-behavioral therapy (CBT), talk therapy, and counseling. These interventions can be beneficial in managing mood fluctuations and mental health issues during menopause.